HEALTHY DIET AUTOPHAGY

&

RENAL DIET

COOKBOOK

2 BOOKS IN 1

TOSHIMORI YOICHI,

MARK DANIEL COOKSEY

AUTOPHAGY

How to Activate your Body and let it Purify
through Water Fasting, Intermittent Fasting,
Keto Diet to Lose Weight, Detox your Body,
Increase Muscle Mass, Slow Down Aging,
Stay Healthy.

TOSHIMORI YOICHI,
MARK DANIEL COOKSEY

Table of Contents

Introduction

This book is about autophagy, which is a gesture or process, in which individuals fast. The individuals that fast they observe marvelous qualities of smartness and agility in them and with the passage of time, the body makes them a big way of combating things. Combating things means that the body is able to endure a lot of pressure while in managerial works and the brain is able to make things look way better than the previous. The book will deal with many aspects of autophagy. What are the qualitative foods that define the working of food and how the activities or daily routine make the working of the body look more effective? The use and routine of autophagy through the intake of diets and how the public is able to get into proper shape will also be contextualized. The use of managerial ways and tactics through which autophagy is easily induced in the body and every deduction that can be affected with time. Therefore, the concept of autophagy and the inter-related concepts of autophagy will be elucidated in this book.

Autophagy can be used to describe a lot of benefits for the people. There are many uses of it. It can be used to cater to skin problems, it can give better improvisations for cancer-related patients, it can give a firm character building by expunging the bad diet from the body, it can also be used to reduce the risk of neuro-related diseases. Autophagy is also a way to make the body level reach the acme of strong blood pressure and all those heart-related diseases are also eliminated through it. Therefore, autophagy has many uses in this regard.

Chapter 1 - What is Autophagy

This chapter will deal with the definition, the working of autophagy, the types of autophagy and the usage of autophagy in the coming time. This chapter will also include the various formations of autophagy through which the people's way is moved forward in the direction. The contextualization of the book is as follows:

Definition

According to Doctor Priya Khorana, the process of autophagy means the exit of food through the stomach and it makes the metabolism look very clean. The cells that are used in this process are easily removed during this process and later there is the rejuvenation of newer cells for healthy growth for the humans. Auto means self and the word phagy means eating. Therefore, autophagy means that the body will eat automatically and with the passage of time, the old food will be removed.

By some authors, it is also related to self-devouring. This is the beneficial omen for your body and the process of self-devouring, the body cells are easily extinguished from the body thoroughly. The process of cellular repair also takes place in this context and the over-all body metabolism reaches its zeal. Thus, the use of cellular repair will make the body look better in the coming. The process of autophagy is a revolutionary self-preserving mechanism that helps in the elimination of carbon-related diseases in the human body.

For some, the definition is also contextualized as the process through which the cells of the body are easily functioned in a better manner. There is also the removal of debris. It is referred to as the process of recycling and removing at the same time. The prolific medical scientist referred to it as the way of resetting your body and the body aims to reach the better part of life. It is also a promotion of better toxin-related concepts of the body and it will amplify the metabolism of the body in a perpetual manner.

Why autophagy works

There is an ancient saying that the body will work if led with a proper mind. The use of autophagy helps to instill a proper mode of management for the people through which the persons are able to lead a happy life. The working of autophagy is also productive because it is able to give marvelous and potential results to the human body. It creates the possibility and creation of better cells that are quite great in their number and they are able to curb strong measurements of disease prevention in them. There are many other benefits of it through which the body is able to receive better quality digestion and heat of hydration. There are numerous working mechanisms that are cultivated in the body through the use of autophagy. Since, the use of autophagy brings about better changes in the human body, therefore, the use of autophagy works in the coming time and it is much effective for the use of the human body.

Autophagy for health

There are five important ways through which autophagy works for the construction of health for the students and civilians. These ways help to restore the health factor for autophagy constructively.

1. Eating a high fat, low carb diet

The eating of a high-fat triggers autophagy in the body. The use of high fat and its gestation ultimately exits some cells from the body through which the people are able to have a better understanding of the body in their dimension. The low carb diet will make your suit for autophagy as the process of elimination of cells will be random in the body and the person will be able to give more value to its body. So, the intake of high fat will make the body have more leniency in it and with the passage of time, the body will get rid of all the cells that make the body look pale and obstructive in the coming time.

2. Go on a protein fast

The autophagy will be helpful for the protein fast. Because in this fast you will be able to do a lot of mass exemption from the body. During the fast of the body, the people will be able to have a better comprehension of the body through which the protein of the body will go away and the body will be given a better way of creating proteins in the coming time. Therefore, going on a protein fast will help to make the body a much better and more regulatory space.

3. Practice Intermittent Fasting

The concept of intermittent fasting is that the body has to take a lot of proteins from the human body and there is a regular break from eating and drinking. There are time intervals through which the body is able to garner more food and water in the body. This time can be used to make the body look better and productive in the coming time. The use of strong fasting can make the body relax and have a sustainable piece of working in the coming. So, if you want to attain a benefit of autophagy of health then do practice intermittent fasting.

4. Exercise Regularly

Exercising regularly can also initiate a fast rate of autophagy for you. The exercising helps to reduce fats allowing for more proteins to actually work in the body. The working of the body helps to maintain a strong pH value of the system and the body is able to foment a healthier metabolism. This is a concept through which the autophagy of the body functions in a better way and with the passage of time, autophagy tends to be sustainable in a better function.

5. Drink a lot of water

Drinking a lot of water also helps you to maintain a stable metabolism of yourself through which you are able to have a yielding understanding of things around. Drinking a lot of water makes the ph value system aware of all the things happening around and with the passage of time, the body is able to make healthier changes in the coming time. Drinking a lot of water will keep the diet clean and healthy and it will make your body fit for any changes coming in the contemporary. Therefore, drinking a lot of water is crucial for you to maintain an autophagy state.

Types of Autophagy

There are three types of autophagy. One is the macro-autophagy, micro-autophagy and chaperone-mediated autophagy.

1. Macro-autophagy

Macro-autophagy is a type of autophagy in which the degradation of organelles occurs. It is a matured vesicle process. It is strongly recommended for the homeostasis process, in which the persons belonging to various paths and parallels are identified in the human being for a perpetual state of mind. The use of macro-autophagy can be illustrated in many ways of the world. The uses are very much in use these days. The use of microautophagy can be related to many uses like the cure of brain diseases and brain coverages. The use of macroautophagy has many abilities embedded in it. It can be used to treat neurodegenerative diseases for the people. The disease-linked aggresomes can be used in many uses to make the fossils and the human platelets working in a better way. The macroautophagy can also be constructed in many ways possible for the people coming forward. Therefore, Macroautophagy is the branch of autophagy, which deals with the process of clearing the established fats in the body.

2. Micro-autophagy

The construct of microautophagy is different from two types of autophagy that are macro and chaperone-mediated autophagy. These autophagias help the micro people and the lysosomal action to be easily overridden by the people and the body state. This practice is adopted by many people abroad and it can also be found with many people and other doctors to be precisely relevant. This practice is very important for the functioning of cells and it helps to give more emphasis to the extermination of diseases in the coming time. Cytoplasmic material is trapped in the cells of the people and the people are able to manifest the uses of autophagy properly. This process is also used for nitrogen deprivation and it can lead to strong illustrations of people effectively. There are three special cases to microautophagy. Micro hexalogy, piecemeal microautophagy and microautophagy of the nucleus. These phages make the body of the human being emerged from the ashes.

There are very important functions of micro-autophagy. There are used for nutrient recycling. This is done for the degradation of lipids. It regulates the composition of the vacuolar membrane. There are many mechanisms of glycogen in it. The pathway that comes through micro-autophagy helps to create a link with the multivesicular bodies, endocytic, membrane proteins and the use of strong organelle size. There is also non-selective micro-autophagy in this regard. There is membrane invagination, vesicle formation, vesicle expansion, vesicle degradation and selective micro-autophagy. These invaginations help to create a better formation of body cells for the persons coming forward and with the passage of time, the body is able to eat all the fats and vitamins of the structure effectively. This practice is of strong use and pertinence and can be regarded effectively in the coming time.

The process of selective micro-autophagy can be observed in all types of eukaryotic cells. This on the other hand is also commonly observed in yeast cells. Therefore, micro-autophagy helps to create a cluster of better engines for the coming community.

3. Chaperone-mediated autophagy

This chaperone-mediated autophagy helps to give more ideas to the process of autophagy. This is referring to the selection of chaperone dependent selection. The selection of soluble proteins is taken in this account. The cytosolic proteins are targeted to lysosomes and directly are related to the concept of lysosome membrane without the requirement of the formation of additional values. The proteins that want to make the structure of CMA are cytosolic proteins and proteins from other compartments. There are some compartments that discuss the nature of CMA and they are worthy to be discussed here. These are the compartments that tend to make the working of the cells more functional and linear in their working. There is selectivity of proteins and the proteins are able to make the manufacture of the engine more compatible. The CMA can be of many uses and regards of the people and the people are able to blend with the work coherently.

The proteins that participate in the CMA are more likely to be engulfed by the main cell of the body. First there is the degradation of cells, there is the presence of cytosolic protein in the making, there is the formation of amino acid in the work, there is lysosome-associated work of the protein type A in the formation, there is a receptor for the membrane of the formation of the work, the two isoforms are found in the cells of the body through which one has to trade genes to the people coming ahead, there are substrates that deal with the process of working for the people and then there are translocation purposes that make the deal of CMA more workable. There is an artificial use of people that do not cater properly to the formation of the work and with the passage of time, there is a better comprehension thing coming forward.

The matter comes to the people of the formation in a close manner and this thing helps to bind the CMA more effectively for the people. Therefore, the use of a close manner can be sorted out more periodically in the coming time. There are some limitations to the CMA process. One is the binding of the substrate of the people coming forward and with the passage of time, the CMA tends to be more linear with time. There are some levels of constraints to the process of CMA as well. With the passage of time, the CMA tends to devolve and if one wants to maintain a proper outlook of CMA then there need to be some limitations. The levels of CMA are easily utilized and they are made under some uncertainties for the people. The people in these uncertainties are not able to proceed with CMA and hence, they are able to come stringently ahead.

These are three types of autophagias discussed above in the effective manner.

Chapter 2 - 9 reasons why autophagy is good for health

This chapter will deal with this discussion about why autophagy is good for health.

1. Autophagy saves your life

As the definition of autophagy has been established above that it is the science in which the body eats its own food so this process can easily save your life effectively. In this process, the eating of fat clearly eliminates the bad food and process that could be hard to tackle while working and with the passage of time, autophagy can bring forth more progress to the people. The autophagy regularities are very effective to handle and they give an enriched benefit while the food is being conserved or stored and with the passage of time, the people are able to learn the advantages of autophagy ultimately.

2. Autophagy improves the length and quality of life

How autophagy improves the length and quality of life, this is a certain assertion needs to be answered. The autophagy people are the people that are confident with their lifestyles, they know what to eat and how to present themselves in front of others and how the improvement is able to be fostered in the coming time. Their body metabolisms make the personality of life much better and they are quite sturdy in their workings coming forward. Therefore, autophagy is able to bolster the length and quality of life in the coming time.

3. Autophagy helps your metabolism work better

The thing about autophagy that cherishes the most is its ability to make the workings better and coherent. The use of autophagy can make the body very lean and effective in its domain and with the passage of time, the people are able to have muscular bodies through it. The metabolism also functions better because of a caring appetite, autophagy has to offer. This caring appetite makes the body completely firm to come forward and with the passage of time, the people are able to have a better relaxation of the time. So, with such benefits, autophagy helps your metabolism to work better.

4. Autophagy helps you to clear out neurodegenerative diseases

The brain is the vibrating and the most important muscle of the body as it governs messages and neutronic transmissions throughout the body. If there are neurodegenerative diseases in the brain and the brain is not able to make proper processions in the body then with the passage of time, the body is able to vacate the diseases effectively. The crux of autophagy is defined to make the brain more adaptable and managerial with the passage of time and thus, the human brain is not able to make any impulsion whatsoever in the coming time. Therefore, autophagy helps you to clear out neurodegenerative diseases.

5. Autophagy helps to regulate inflammation

The process of autophagy is also essential while maintaining a level of inflammation in the body. The process is all found in the founding of the body through which the body reduces the risk of noises in the coming. The inflammation is the increase in blood pressure and with a special piece of autophagy fast forward, the people are able to make things more effective for their bodies. This is the autophagy that one needs to understand in the coming and the inflammation is all pertinent for the body to come. Therefore, autophagy is much useful for inflammation to come in line.

6. Autophagy helps us find infectious diseases regularly

Autophagy is also very effective when it comes to fighting infectious diseases. The body engine is designed in such a length through which the body is able to make devoid of things effectively. The infectious diseases that make the bodies more workable will be used in this regard. The autophagy will make the body length much lean and cooperative and with the passage of time, the body is able to nurture effectively in the coming. Therefore, autophagy is more complacent for you when it comes to fight infectious diseases regularly.

7. Autophagy also improves muscle performance

How muscle performance is improved this needs to be discussed here in detail. Muscles are used to make more time in the coming and they are built on certain vascular tissues that are round in their shape. Muscles get rusted if there is no proper use of a keto diet and proper intake of carbo related diet in the muscles and with the passage of time, the muscles need to be in a better linear order than before. So, the use of autophagy is also helpful in making muscle performance more compatible and lenient in its design.

8. Autophagy helps prevent cancer loss

Autophagy helps to control cancer brewing in the human body. It prevents cancer from further burgeoning in the human body and with the passage of time, the human body is able to supplement strong things compatibly. It can also control genome stability and can improve the working DNA more coherently. The risk of cancer is easily controllable when it comes to the induction of autophagy in it. The research process will be highly appreciable for the coming tasks of the world and the people will be able to apply with the passage of time. The crux of autophagy will help the patients to come evolving with time and the people will learn things more compatibly and ferociously.

9. Autophagy improves digestion health

The process of autophagy is very material for the use of health. It helps to give better stamina, stable mental systems and the use of effective neutronic systems that can make the body immune to diseases. It can lower the ph value with a possible rate of affection and with the passage of time, the community is able to learn things in a much better and compatible manner. The platform of autophagy can further nourish many creative aesthetics for the body and so with the passage of time, the body will be able to improve health systematically.

10. Autophagy improves your skin health

Once you are eating things in an effective manner, you are actually making a better overview of your skin effectively. The idea here is very simple, that is you have to come up with splendid assertions that can make the body look more effective in the coming. The skin gets all right and great with the passage of time and you are able to witness the portfolio of yourself holistically. Therefore, the process of autophagy is very resourceful for the public and the people can learn a lot for the coming time.

11. Autophagy may support a healthy weight

Autophagy requires a fat eating process. The fats, lipids and proteins all are very healthy for the coming time and with the process of time, autophagy is able to inculcate a better process of stamina building in you. The use of strong weight and proper digestion helps you to make things turn around in a systematic manner and with the passage of time, your muscles become rigid and you become more and more reflective in their time.

12. Autophagy minimizes self-death of cells

The regeneration of cells is an important aspect through which people are able to form multiple dimensions in the coming time. The edifice of autophagy helps to minimize the death of cells in the human being and the people are able to create better understandings of their body respectively. Therefore, the minimization of dead cells is found using autophagy.

Chapter 3 - How Autophagy works

This chapter will talk about the working of autophagy that how it comes with respect to time.

The basics

Autophagy has described above is a self-digesting mechanism of the human body. It involves the formation of a double-membrane vesicle through which the individual is able to see the fats of the body go in depletion. This process is also used to add the encapsulation of cytoplasm and other materials in an evolving manner with the passage of time. There are sixteen level autophagy protein involved in this manner. These systems produce modified complexes of autophagy regulators. There is the process of nucleation and completion of autophagias formation and then it is used to fuse it with lysosomes. There are two processes that are required in this scenario and with the passage of time, the people are able to make huge benefits through it. In mammals there are proteins that tend to deal with it.

The elongation also occurs in the process of autophagy where the people are able to have a better version of things coming with the passage of time. There is a kinase activity that is required in this process through which the individuals are harbor better credentials of the things required in the process. Atg 13, Atg 1 and Atg 2 were easily associated with the remark. All these autophagy proteins require the formation of many other instruments in a proper fashion in this regard. The elongation has the combination of two ubiquitin conjugation materials in this regard. It remains bound to the autophagosome membrane until some of it is easily bonded to the membrane. As soon as autophagous formation is completed, the Atg 16, Atg 32 and Atg 5 are there to recognize things in an appropriate manner. Now the completed autophagosome is ready for fusion with the end of the molecules and with the passage of time, the people are able to have a better understanding of the process.

The process of autophagy regulation is adamant to make the metabolism of the body more adaptable and the basics are enough for the body to undergo a positive change in themselves.

Insulin also regulates autophagy in the human body. These moments of autophagy will always be up to the mark of other people coming forward and the people, who come under the pressure of bad working as an insult so therefore, it is necessary to understand that how the formation of autophagy comes forward and it can come with many possible directions in the coming.

Mutations of many other autophagy-related ingredients for the prospect of better metabolism and health factor. There is a damage regulated autophagy modulator that tries to deal with the assertion of making the fats level descend with the passage of time. There is a manner in which the death level of the organisms is raised to death and the cell organisms are able to make the people go with positive sway. The p 53 committed cell membrane helps to make body level very mature with the passage of time and the people are able to induce much more betterment in the body. There is chromatin remodeling and the persons are able to induce more and more enrichments with the passage of time.

Macroautophagy

This is a type of autophagy. The autophagy will give immense pleasure to the cell bodies that are functioning well in the body. This is the type of autophagy that will give a clear perception of things coming in the letdown process and it kills the process of cell destruction easily. This is autophagy, which usually gives many deprivations to the body but with the passage of time, it evolves the body to a stable state.

Micro-autophagy

This autophagy involves the use of cellular disintegration which can be very healthy for the human body.

Chaperone mediated autophagy

This is the evolved process of autophagy and macro-autophagy.

Other types of autophagy

As per scientific evidence, there is no other use of autophagy required to illustrate. But there is more emphasis to bone autophagy

Autophagy used in other therapeutic agents

Autophagy is used in therapeutic agents to cure neurogenic agents.

Chapter 4 - Stimulating autophagy

In this chapter the stimulation of autophagy will be approached.

Fasting

Fasting needs to be done in order to observe the advantages of autophagy. Following meat plans need to be followed.

1. Black and white Pudding

This pudding has a fixed amount of cream in it that is used as a dessert in all the foods and can be re-created on many festivals and food. It is organic in its nature and can be created in a very short span of time. It is very fresh and a lot of customers want to have a taste of it once they have done eating their regular meals.

2. Ginger Bread Biscuits

Gingerbread biscuits are widely celebrated in all parts of the world and they are eaten with full relish as well. These biscuits are very keen on their core as they tend to be very fresh and are consumed on a daily amount of basis. The gingerbread biscuits are present in all prices and ranges for the customers that want to eat it. They are affordable in their limits.

3. Liquor Chocolates

Liquor chocolates are very delicious and they have a taste of liquor in them, which adds a taste of acidity in them. The amount of liquor is very fresh for the body as it easily gives a fresh tone of digestion to the body. There is less heat generated in the body while drinking it and it can be very helpful at times for many festivals. It is important to have a healthy diet these days and if liquor chocolates are used as a means to get to the balanced chart then they must utilize it at all costs.

4. Chicken made with a stuffing of fruits and vegetables

Chicken, which is made with a lot of acidic strains, if it is combined with a stuffing of fruits and vegetables; then it can be very ketogenic for the consumers. The process is very healthy for the people and it ensures all the strong amounts of protein intake that humans can vitalize. This is the ability of chicken mixed with vegetables that can be very helpful for the individuals.

5. Haggis

It is a stomach of sheep, which is embedded with oatmeal and offal. This oatmeal and offal can be very effective for the metabolism of the individuals as it produces a great range of intakes for the people. There is a residue of acidic strains and ketogenic inputs that give the customer a relishing tone to digest. It is made with proper care and intellect and can be further assessed for many benefits. It is not only available in Scotland but can be retrieved also in other countries. This is a better provision for the customers, which gives it proper digestion and intake.

6. Dumpling Soup

The dumpling soup is revered by the doctors to be very helpful at the present age. A lot of people whether living in the west or the east are consuming a lot of amount of ketogenic and acidic diet for their daily usage. This intake creates an acidic heat in the body and in this way the dumpling soup caters to this dilemma with full urge and discipline. What happens is that the moment the soup is entrained into the windpipe of the human; the body system becomes very energetic. Hence, the dumpling soup is able to get a lot of help for the human body and it is also recommended by many.

7. Toshikoshi Soba

Toshikoshi Soba is a Japanese dish that can easily deal with the autophagy of the body. It is baked using a ketogenic powder that can be very helpful for the consumers. It has a spread of noodles all around it that can give an acidic taste as well. It is for all the consumers and individuals that want a balanced diet in their bodies and it can turn around to be very effective and helpful to the local people. It is affordable by a layman throughout Japan and it has fresh ingredients that are recommended for the body.

8. Latkes

If you want a ketogenic diet that has fresh vegetables and juices, then you must refer to latkes. It is an Israeli diet that has all the fresh ingredients that your body can use and you can come up with a healthy amount of taste for it. All you need is to develop a mindset in your body that you want to achieve the best of you. There are crispy potato chips engraved in it and there can be more possibilities in it as well. You can have the entire taste and relish of it. Just buy it near any store and you will achieve the best of your health as well.

9. Puerto Rican Pasteles

Puerto Rican Pasteles is the famous dish that is available in Puerto Rico and it can be very fresh for the public over there. It is made with raisins, olives, pork, and fish. The tamales that are made are frozen first and then they are served to their customers. The reason for their freezing is because they can be well served while they are frozen. The pastels are also very affordable for all the customers located in various parts of the world and there are many special features of them. They can be curated in all sizes and demands.

10. Carmela

If you are a vegetarian and are avoiding chicken meats to be all lean and ketogenic then this cabbage-made dish is the real deal for you. You have to be very cautious while eating as its single intake can be very heavy. Not only cabbage but it has a slight amount of chicken ginger folds that can be very helpful for digestion. Therefore, it is important to have a balanced diet on holiday and this diet is recommended by all the prodigies to be of supreme relish.

11. Jansson's Temptation

This dish is very delicious and it starts with a tempting scotch of potato casserole and cream herring. This temptation compels the customer to it and there are many positive reviews about it in the country. Family and middle-class men all are enjoying it and they require a lot of usage for it. Also, this dish comes in all prices and ranges and there are many varieties to it as well.

12. Carp

This carp has a special amount of green leaves decorated at its sides and it can be used to access the food regime of human metabolism. The autophagy that is produced by this dish is very instrumental in its making and it provides all the comfort levels that can be used to get a hydrated amount of autophagy in it. The carp creates a sense of relish in the human body and due to it; it allows the person to grow more diet tactics. You can easily be healthy and fresh throughout your routine.

13.   Mince Pie

This dish of England has its own taste to check and one can easily afford the autophagy in his body through it. The diet of the human body is very important to be maintained on holidays and this mince pie can be the real deal for the humans. The mince pie has a sweet touch to it that makes the customer very happy about it.

14.   Yebeg Wot

This is a Christmas dish that has a very good reputation worldwide. It is created by giving a soft lamb pouring all around it. This Wot is spread with flatbread and it can be very helpful for the eaters to have fun for it.

15.   Tamales

These tamales are portable corn husk rolls that can be very instrumental for the diet appetite. These are present in all names and sizes and can be effective in all ins and outs. They are presentable in all fruits, vegetables, and cheeses.

16.   Mashed Potatoes

The last recipe to this list is mashed potatoes. These potatoes are very instrumental in their making and they have to be boiled and peeled to see how they are formed. They are mashed in a proper way to attract the customers and they have an attractive lure all around them.

Therefore, these are the food and diets that can be used to celebrate in different parts of the world. They are celebrated and adored all around the world. People come from all the places to see the attraction, the taste and the uniqueness of these dishes. They are used to induce autophagy in the human body.

While fasting following foods needs to be avoided at all costs.

1.   Sugary Drinks

Sugar is a dangerous product and a demanding food recipe. It can be sweet and at the same time, it can require a lot of sweat to be removed from the body. All those drinks like the Pepsi drinks and the hydrated drinks that have an amount of sugar in them are too difficult to be removed from the day that the human body has to do a lot of grueling exercise for them. Also, the blood vessels that get in contact with the sugar streamline are two exposed to collapse because these sugar particles tend to disturb the vessels of the human body. Furthermore, the sugary drinks also disturb the healthy metabolism of the body and also they make the routine of the body very lazy. Therefore, the sugary drinks need to be avoided at all cost to stay healthy and fit.

2. Pizzas

Pizzas carry a lot of calorie and chemical products that are able to make you fat and lazy. These pizzas always create a source of relish for the individuals but nobody knows what happens in the latter. Pizzas have to be eaten but there needs to be a systematic kind of balance while they are being consumed. The dairy products, the cheese, and the bread all are able to create a lot of fat tendencies among the individuals that eat it. Thus, it is mandatory for people to realize the plight of this fast food. Otherwise, it can be very detrimental to the public.

3.   White Bread

Although white bread is considered to be very healthy for the individuals in the morning; but it also has some detrimental qualities as well. White bread contains a vicious amount of calories that can raise the blood level of humans. It is also the real reason behind the vast emergence of heart strokes in the patients. Therefore, it is important to take a minimum amount of bread in the morning. Also, there is an alternative to this dairy product as well. The brown bread can be used as an alternative as it carries a lesser amount of calories in it.

4. Industrial Vegetable Oils

Industrial vegetable oils are very acidic in nature. They carry a lot of calories, fat oils and other dairy ingredients in them. There are also added fats in them that tend to create a lot of hurdles for body metabolism. Their intake can create troubles in blood clotting and it can also be the reason for heart attacks. Industrial vegetable oils are very precarious for health. They all can be very haunting for the consumers; there needs to be minimum use of vegetable oils for cooking recipes.

5. Margarine

Margarine is presumed to be like butter but it has many cancerous ingredients to it. Margarine possesses all the important components of butter like amino acids, fats, and lipids, which can cause a urinary impact on the body. It is, therefore, very important that the use of margarine be minimized at all costs.

The alternative to this product can be the use of butter as it has minimum calories in it.

6.   Pastries, cookies, and cakes

We all like to eat a lot of pastries and cookies because we get attracted to their odor and taste. They have the variety that qualifies for our interest and we like to stuff our bellies with a lot of pastries just for the moment of fun. However, we do not know that these cakes and pastries have calorie content that is very enjoyable for us. But fewer people know that they create stubborn fat in our bellies that require a lot of effort and exercise to let it go. Also, they are the primary reason for a lazy routine and if their consumption is kept forward then they will reduce the ketogenic process of the body.

7.   French Fries.

If you think that you want to obese in a short span or want to win a fat body competition, then potato fries and French fries are the real deal for you. Without their intake, you cannot be fat. Although this statement donates a connotation that the fries are good but their storage can lead to the rise of many inflammatory diseases in the human body. They also have a profuse amount of calorie intake in their body and thus, can make you look lazy. The acidity in your body can rise to its acme if the accumulation of French fries is taken in your body.

8. Agave Nectar

Agave nectar contains a large amount of fructose in the body that can yield a lot of sweetness in your blood. This sweetness can compact your vessels and make your metabolism become dull and void. Also, kidney fractures and other bodily malfunctions come in your body and you can get the worst amount of digestion in no time. So the intake of agave nectar is not good for your body and you must try your best in making the less of it.

9. Low Fat Yogurt

Yogurt is a healthy product, which is very supplementary for your health. It has a relevant of dairy ingredients that boost activeness and agility in you. You get a fresh start to your routine if you are able to muster up usage. There is a minimum amount of fat stored in it as well. However, low-fat yogurt is not good as it contains an obsess amount of yogurt that could be detrimental for you. It has profuse lipids that can make your face look pale in no time and it can be also quite dangerous to store in the belly. Instead of it, one should go for the full-fat yogurt that has good calorie content for you and you can feel all fresh and great for it. The low-fat yogurt can be put to the fermentation process and its fermentation can yield an enormous amount of protein for you.

10. Ice cream

Ice cream is used as a dessert for many but it has a great number of calories stored in it. It comes in all flavors and like the other acidic foods mentioned above, it can lead to proper storage of fats in your body. Also, the biscuit content that is present below the ice-cream has a huge number of calories in it and thus, the ice cream is a fat creating package for you. You can make a great alternative to this menace by creating better ice cream. For creating the better version of ice cream, mature ingredients need to be used for better results.

11. Candy Bars

If you want to carry a short snack with you that can create a fatty metabolism in you, then candy bars are the real menace to be blamed. Created with a touch of candy, flavored with sugar and coated with chocolates; these ingredients reflect the highest amount of acidity in your body. They boost calorie content in you. They create fat storages in you and they do not let to go away in a jiffy. They have a lot of bars of accumulation in their creation and they all are very haunting for you. Thus, it is important that candy bars are pertinent to be stayed away from and their intake can damage your cholesterol level as well.

12.   Processed Meat

Meat is the highest amount of protein giver than any other food. However, processes meat needs to be finished by all means possible. Because it has all the chemical ingredients that trigger fat accumulation in your body and it is very dampening for human metabolism as well. It is also not covered in healthy packing and it gives a sheer amount of negativity in your body as well. The meat further destroys the good quality of chlorine in your body and you are not able to regain the advantages of a balanced diet in a sensible way.

13. Processed Cheese

Processed cheese is filled with filler ingredients that completely eradicate protein and healthy fats in your body. On the contrary, regular cheese is very fine for the body as the content of food is compatible with your body. Therefore, the idea of processed cheese is not good for your body as it destroys the healthy metabolism of the body.

14. Veggie Petties

Veggie Petties are very good for health but their procession can also be very daunting for the human body. The vegetables that are used in these sandwiches have a chlorine-deficit in it and can not be used as a healthy regimen. Because chlorine impacts your blood and having a chlorine-deficit diet can make you feel tired and can boost you in becoming a lazy person. Also, it can accumulate a vast amount of fats in the body. You are not able to feel fresh when you eat a lot of veggie patties. You are not able to get the quality of intake of freshness in the body and thus, you end up being fat and there is a massive increase of cholesterol in the body.

15.   Packaged Turkey

Turkey has an abundance of sodium and proteins in it but a package of it is not able to give the amount of balanced diet that you want. Its packaging is very detrimental for your level and you end up becoming very unhygienic throughout the year. You can either buy less sodium in the package or you will end up being lazy and feel very unhealthy. Thus, packaged turkey is a good diet but not a ketogenic diet to eat.

16.   Energy Bars

These energy bars are hailed to be energy bars but you are not able to achieve an energy full diet because of it. The energy bars are not able to give an important intake of proteins as well. According to Dr. Garwis, protein bars are all just processed chemicals. And also, they have a lot of chemicals embedded in them. They are chemical creators that do not give enough health to the individuals and they are able to a sustained metabolism rate for the individuals.

17. Bran Muffins

This recipe can be a quick breakfast diet but actually, it leaves a lot of calories especially for the individuals, who consume it. It has a profuse chemical of sugar, formaldehyde, wheat, and flour and they all try their best to creating fats in themselves.

18. Multigrain Bread

This bread has the sugar embedded chemical in it that can be harmful to your body if taken massively. It is assumed to be very healthy as it has a multi-grain fiber attached to it but overall, it required a lot of wheat and sugar in it, which can be detrimental for you. It can also spike the blood sugar level in you and you will feel remorseful while you are eating it.

19.   Flavored Oatmeal

Well, do you think that you can find any faults in regular oatmeal when it is served in front of you; because it has everything that the body required? However, research is proved that oatmeal tends to boost massive calories in you as it has a lot of sodium and sugar-related chemicals staked in it. Also, the creamy flavor fosters fats and chemicals in yourself and can be very dangerous for you as well.

20.   Reduced-Fat Peanut Butter

The reduced-fat peanut butter is very good for breakfast or even regular lunch meals. It has a reduced amount of sodium intake in it and contains fewer fats comparatively. They are naturally created with the fermentation process of the sugar. However, they have one strong drawback. That is that they have to be energy deficit and they can bring more fats in the bodies due to reduced-fat peanut butter.

21.   Couscous

Couscous might be a vital grain to feast but it is just like pasta because it is very dangerous in its making. Couscous want to build the massive intake of autophagy in you and you want it for any reason. However, the sugar and sodium level in couscous is very high and at some level, it can be very dangerous for you as well.

Therefore, these foods are not good for the body intake as they dampen the healthy figments of the body and try to impede positive metabolism in the body. The damage that these ingredients due to their bodies are very obscene and there must be the use of super-foods that can heal the body with full zeal.

So, in fasting the aforementioned foods need to be avoided and used accordingly.

Dieting

While dieting, do your best to make the best out of you and eat the following foods.

1. Kelp

Kelp is a portion of fresh green food that boosts iodine intake in the body. It is also rich in calcium, magnesium, and potassium, which can be very supplemental for the body. The intake of kelp should be very moderate to give the body a nominal control of its care. The green ingredients reduce fat and terrible amino acids that could be harmful to the body. Also, the love handles that are created on the sides of the stomach are easily rectified with full zeal and energy.

2. Ginger

Ginger is very useful in treating arthritis and can very suitable for healthy digestion as well. It is recognized worldwide for its ability to treat nausea and it has been doing it in a spectacular way.

3. Mushrooms

There are many types of mushrooms that can cater to healthy digestion in the body. The types include a white button, shiitake, portabella, and cremini. These mushrooms also lower the cholesterol level in the body and create a ketogenic state of digestion in the human body. These mushrooms are easy to cook and eat and apart from healing benefits, they can be used in desserts as well.

4. Beets

Beets contain a plethora of many supplements for the body. They give carbs, calcium, iron, vitamin a and vitamin c. These vitamins are very helpful for the body as they regenerate a lot of energy for the body to do work. Many people in the contemporary world are pursuing beets for the gain of carbohydrates. Beets are easy to buy and afford and can be able to give outstanding performances in the human body.

5. Probiotics

First, let us understand what are probiotics? Probiotics are the microorganisms that attack germs entering your body and they are very useful in making you aloof of diseases. They are very tiny in their chemistry that can be found in yogurt, kefir and soy beverages. These probiotics can also be obtained in many other products as well. These probiotics can be used to treat irritable bowel syndrome, skin infections, and certain cancers.

6.   Swiss Chard

This chard provides a huge amount of source for vitamins c,e, and k for the human body. It also gives fiber, zinc, and calcium. The chard is also available in a variety of leaf colors. The taste is the combination of salty and bitter. This nutrition-packed vegetable must be supporting bone health; fights stress-related disease and also have the anti-inflammatory disease to cater as well.

7.   Aloe Vera

Aloe Vera is a curing herb that is used to heal facial scars and also cater to the digestion burns in the body. The digestion that is due to an acidic diet creates burning conditions in the body and the intake of aloe vera can also provide healthy minerals for the body. It is found in almost every price and variation. It has an anti-inflammatory nature in it and it attacks all the inflammatory diseases that can be precarious for the body. A bio-mediating form is also present in the core of Aloe Vera that tries to provide better compensation for the results in a human body. Also, this herb specialized in curing the headache of the body and tries its best to create a moderate form in the body. Aloe vera has all the proper chemical ingredients that can create sustenance of the entire human system. Therefore, aloe vera is a healthy herb that is very helpful for the body to heal.

There are many spiritual lessons apparent in Aloe Vera as well. Coming from healing, herb relaxes the system of the mental coordination of a human body and the human being, who is taking the herb comes into an emotional connection with the herb. The herb transcends its healing qualities to humans at all cost and there is no hurdle of its extraction.

8. Apple Cider Vinegar

Apple Cider Vinegar is a curing herb that gives all the relaxation to the human body. It is very efficient in pro-biotics that can cure the mindset of the tensed human body and it can also yield proper salvation to the human body as well. This Apple Cider is usually not found in any other product rather than green herbs and it has many other probiotics that yield safety for the humans.

9. Lemons

Lemons are very healthy for the human metabolism. It has enriched zinc components in it that carve a spectacular body in the human structure. The digestion becomes very easy and no reverting into the esophagus is done in such a scenario. Therefore, the intake of lemons can be very helpful for the human body to enjoy and it is a total package for the human body to enjoy. Also, throat scratches and burns can be easily healed using the lemonade, which yet again is the component of lemon.

Exercising

For exercising, you have to do regular physical exercise along with minute level weight training.

Chapter 5 - Water fasting and ketosis diet

Water fasting and ketosis diet helps to maintain a better place of autophagy in your body. The meals required for water fasting are as follows:

Extended Water fasting

1. Tomatoes

Tomatoes are the best ketogenic foods one can possibly have. It has many nutrients in it. Tomatoes are a great source of Vitamin c. They also provide Vitamin B6. You can have a tomato and then can use it in your favorite salad as well. Therefore, it is an enriched supplement that provides you a ketogenic diet.

2. Almonds

If you want to have a quick ketogenic supplement, then an almond can serve the best purpose to you. They are composed of high fats and can be easily used to store a good amount of energy in you. Also, there is no grueling amount of energy required while its consumption.

3. Spinach

The leafy vegetable, which is green in color is very good for health. It is also very versatile in nature. Spinach can yield the best amount of taste for the public as it verily recommended by all the medical experts. If you want a fresh ketogenic breakfast, then spinach is the real deal for you.

4. Parsley

Parsley is a ketogenic food that is rich in autophagy. It can be used for various purposes as well. It can be used to cleanse the kidney level and can be used in curbing heat digestion. You can also use its variety in many ways to make your food look good.

5. Jalapeno

For a healthy ketogenic diet, the jalapeno is very crucial for health. Jalapeno can be used in many ways and tactics to get to know the autophagy of the body. This ketogenic supplement can support the endocrine system as well.

6. Avocado

If you are a bodybuilder and want to assume yourself to be the next big thing in the world then you surely have to try avocado. This supplement is the powerhouse for you. If you use it properly then certainly you can achieve all the healthiness and agility, you want in your body.

7. Basil

Basil is an amazing ketogenic supplement that is designed to boost energy in your bodies. It is composed of a scientific chain of carbohydrates that ensures anti-inflammation in your body. It is available in all pieces and products anywhere in the shop. It is very quick to eat and it has all the products to be ensured. Therefore, it is important for the supplements to be taken properly and in order to be ketogenic in nature, the supplement basil can be arranged systematically.

8.   Dark Lettuces

If you are missing the fantastic dark lettuces for your ketogenic diet then you are committing the worst blunder of your life. You have to try this ingredient as it will enormous health benefits and the only way you are able to reap its benefits is that you understand its mechanism at all costs. It has a deep color of minerals in it. The color indicates special vitamins for your body like vitamin c and vitamin k. The green pigment includes chlorophyll in your body and you can end up being very fresh in your daily routine.

9.   Celery

This is a great alkalizing food for many reasons. It has a huge amount of water in it. It has vitamins like c and k. The composition is filled with electrolytes that can provide health to your body in no time. This ketogenic also reduces high blood pressure. This food can be easily chopped and diced anywhere and can be presentable in all forms and sizes. The cream of celery is also very great for you in all regards.

10.   Carrots

Carrot is a favorite ketogenic food for many. IT has all the potential vitamins in it that can be used with full zeal and glory. Vitamins like A and C are present in a massive amount. You can also use them in your fruit juices like the green juice. You can also roast them in many ways possible and they can serve as an excellent model of decoration for your barbecue. However, not a lot more cooking must be there because a lot of cooking can make the food very acidic. There are sweet potatoes and orange winter squash that is used in many dishes for you. The rosemary roasted carrots, the curry-spiced carrots, and spiced carrots can be helpful in any desire or circumstance.

11.   Sea Vegetables

Sea vegetable serves as excellent recipes and supplements when you want to serve yourself with autophagy . It is rich in magnesium, calcium, and sodium. It is embedded with vitamins. Vitamins like A, C and K. They are basically eaten in a macrobiotic diet for this purpose. Sea veggies are also popular to have an ocean-like flavor, though they make tasty additions and salads as well. Nori wraps are a very excellent replacement for grain-based wraps.

12.   Sprouted Almonds

Almonds are a great choice for alkalizing and they need a proper mechanism to be used properly. The soaking and sprouting even have many benefits. It has many vitamins like E and C. Almonds are great vegan protein and fiber also. If you use these sprouted almonds in a homogeneous mixture then these provide anti-inflammation in no time.

13. Bok Choy

This healthy diet is capable of transforming many diets for your body. This bok choy is packed with vitamin k and c. It is very rich in antioxidants and is very cancerous for other persons as well. You can add these bok choys to soups and can give more salads and wraps in it as well. There is a simple baby bok choy, sweet and spicy bok choy, and Korean bok choy.

14. Raw Pumpkin Seeds

This beautiful supplement can be very effective for the health regime. These seeds leave ketogenic ash in the blood when they are eaten in the body. They make the body more ketogenic and purer when they are in the body and hence, these are raw in their desires as well. They have a high amount of chlorophyll in their pigments due to which the circulation of the human body is more agile and fast. They are also a great source of iron and protein.

They also make a sweet crunch for your desserts as well.

15. Pink Sea Salt

The Himalayan salt has a very spree of benefits for its consumers. This salt has over eighty-four percent of minerals like magnesium, potassium, and calcium. This salt can cure headaches, joint pain, and fatigue and muscle issues. If you know what to do with the salt then you can easily buy and purchase it. You just need to consume it raw and then you can reap all the benefits of it.

16. Matcha Green Tea

The green tea is not like the regular green tea it has a great amount of nutrition for you. It is not heated or processed like any other tea and if you are able to think of other raw food then this is the prime tea. This tea has an abundance of chlorophyll in it and it has many bodily effects as well. It can improve mood and contains less caffeine for you and other acidic ingredients in it. It also has a great amount of calming effect on your body. If you want to start a great amount of breakfast in your day then this matcha green tea is the next big thing for you.

17. Spirulina

You want to have sea algae that can be very fantastic for your blood flow and if you are searching for such then spirulina is the next big thing for you. The nutrition of this diet is very healthy for your body. IT has, in it, four grams of protein that can be very captivating for your body. It is also packed with vitamin A and can give you a lot of other minerals as well.

There is no hectic amount of researching for it and you have to be very decent while searching for it. You can try it other smoothies as well. You may try it in Raspberry and Blue Spirulina Smoothie. Therefore, these kinds of diets can give you a lot of energy and relish in you for a quality of relaxation in it. Spirulina is also affected by a large amount of spiritualization that can very impact-full in this scenario.

Thus, these are the alkalizing supplements that provide enriched healthy metabolic systems to the bodies and the bodies grow exactly in all sizes and forms due to these. The supplements are carefully examined and they are attained in all costs and packages for the consumers. They generate a high rate of water fasting in you.

Ketogenic diet

The Ketogenic diet and how it works

Are you fat and looking for a planned diet to be lean and fit? Does your corporate lifestyle impede you're eating habits and does not make you feel fresh or energetic? Or simply you do not have the time to research for a balanced diet? If any of these questions bother you then I believe that you are reading the right book at the moment. This book believes in the quality of the diet and prioritizes it over-exercise. The ketogenic diet is the real answer, your obscene mind is looking for and if you apply it then yes, the big tummy of yours will be easily overridden.

The ketogenic diet has natural working. It is composed of such fruits and products that have a ketogenic PH value. This value minimizes the presence of fat and dairy products and allows you to stay healthy throughout your routine. Before, we delve what is the ketogenic diet? Let us examine what is meant by the ketogenic diet. The ketogenic diet is the diet, which has a chemical composition of fruits that have a PH value of above 7 and they are generally water-based in their chemicals. Meaning is that they have enriched quantities of hydrogen and oxygen items in them that become very sustainable for the human body to function. The ketogenic diet fruits contain oranges, mangoes, tomatoes, seeds, legumes, and tofu. In case of a heavy diet and hectic routine, we humans always want to be lean and active and if we fill our stomachs with fast food then we cannot be proactive. Hence, we need a diet that is aloof of all these fats and lipids and can sustain a healthy metabolism throughout our routine.

The working of the ketogenic diet is very progressive in its nature. It is composed of a ketogenic diet regime, which has the theory about it. The theory states that the food molecules, in a ketogenic diet, can be so pure in their PH core that they can prevent harmful diseases from occurring to the human body. This book will not delve into such controversies but would advocate the proper use of the ketogenic diet for the betterment of the human body. So, the chemical composition of a ketogenic diet is based on acidic ash and ketogenic ash. These two components are produced through various biomechanical experiments that yield potential for the people. Ketogenic ash is produced by fruits and vegetables that are green in color and have a ketogenic PH value. The liquid that is used for the synthesis of a ketogenic diet is the residue of the citrus food and acts to give a sumptuous touch to the diet.

Once a ketogenic diet is produced, it is used by consumers to prevent their feeble bodies from the dose of attack of kidney stones and heart diseases. The fruits, once they digested, they help to make the metabolism of the body very ketogenic in a natural way. No amount of burping or fat storage is apparent after the consumption of a ketogenic diet. The diet of food saves a lot of time of consumption and erases any unnecessary fat, which is being stored in the body. In this way, the working of having a ketogenic diet is very nice and it could be able the easy way to be fit. Also, working has many advantages. First and foremost, it builds a solid muscle mass, which is able to make the body look very attractive and strong. A healthy body structure can allow the body to go away in all ifs and buts. Researchers have published their study about the ketogenic diet in the journal, named as Osteoporosis International. They state that many bodybuilders also tend to use the ketogenic diet for their own benefit. Diseases like diabetes, chronic kidney disease, and cardiovascular disease can be cured and also it is meant to cure the fractured fabric in humans resulting as an outcome of sports in humans. Therefore, the major idea of a ketogenic diet is to eat fruits and vegetables and drink lemon-lime as all these components are ketogenic in nature.

Once you have done the intake of a ketogenic diet, you will feel very fresh and great. The pigments that are present in the upper surfaced of the foods give comforting digestion in your large intestine. You are not able to feel any heat burn or issues while you are intaking the ketogenic diet and thus, in no time, you are able to come close to a balanced diet. Therefore, working of the very natural ketogenic diet, calm and clean for your body.

According to scientists, autophagy can also be achieved by creating a fixed amount of diet intakes in the body. The scientists believe that if you are able to carve out a splendid moment for your appetite then this means you are actually pursuing a ketogenic diet. Therefore, it is important to understand that a fixed amount of nutrition can be very effective for your body intake and can yield success for you in no time.

The Amazing Benefits of a ketogenic diet

Do you want to be stable in your health regime and eat fresh things simultaneously? Do you think you need to know the proper diet of your regime while working and sleeping? If you want to achieve a healthy food routine, then the ketogenic diet is the real deal for you. In the previous chapters, we had discussed the alluring notions of a ketogenic diet and now, we will look into the amazing benefits of it.

First and foremost is the sheer activeness that a person tends to achieve while he is eating a ketogenic diet. He feels healthy and looks healthy and wants to be doing a lot of things while he is having a ketogenic diet. He can think properly and can get rid of inflammatory diseases that can cause him suffering. He has a strong discipline that can be navigated in any way possible and thus, he is the next big thing for his users. Also, the longevity of life in this scenario and truly, a ketogenic diet can do a lot of wonders for the individual. Therefore, a ketogenic diet has a lot to do for the fitness and active-ness in the human body.

If you want to look green and fresh on your face, then the ketogenic diet can be very helpful in this regard. Studies show that the ketogenic diet is very popular in making a healthy face for you. The number of herbs and breakfast recipes you have for yourself, up-bring a good amount of freshness on your face as well on your skin. Thus, autophagy is very crucial for having great skin and face.

Ketogenic diet protects bone density and muscle mass. The mineral intake that you get after having a ketogenic diet can protect your bone density. The bones need certain minerals that are used to cure the excessive number of hurdles one gets while running. The minerals are given by the ketogenic diet and you are able to get a stronger bone for life. If you are a bodybuilder and want to reap the benefits of the bone then you have to accumulate more ketogenic foods in you that can be very beneficial for you. For example, muscle mass can be secured in an acute manner if you tend to get more and more almonds and other ketogenic foods. You have to be very lenient when you are having the ketogenic diet because the benefit of a ketogenic diet like the muscle mass and the bone density will be instrumental for you. Just always look at the bright side of the diet and you will feel very productive while you do it.

In today's world, tensions are like a haunting disease that wants to remain at your back for no reason. Everywhere you go, you get a tertiary level of tension. There is the tension of graduating, the tension of succeeding in life, the tension of getting a job and the tension of whatnot. You believe that the tension can be very successive for you but in the latter, it turns out to be adverse. Scientists have claimed medical drugs for its cure but the only reasonable cure is the use of a ketogenic diet. The enzymes that you get through vegetables lower the risk of your hyper blood tension and then you can achieve all the relish of your lifestyle in no time. Also, your blood level starts to resonate with full capacity and you will feel like a superman every place you go, therefore; hypertension and tensed matters get an upper hand of resolution when you get to know the prospect of a ketogenic diet.

You are able to get a lot of chronic pains in your body due to many reasons. You get to the bottom of any problem; you solve it and end up having chronic pain in your body. Chronic pain refers to any tertiary amount of pain in your body and you are able to get to the harmfulness of it in no time. Therefore, chronic pain is the most devastating headache that you can get and the only effective cure of it is the ketogenic diet. Yes, the ketogenic diet is very important for you to maintain as the blood level minimizes when lemon or other ketogenic water is induced in the body. So, this is another benefit of a ketogenic diet and it does not matter if you are a walker, a boxer or even a corporate worker, you must have a ketogenic diet in you if you wish to give all that you crave.

Recipes in a ketogenic diet

Breakfast recipes

If you want to start afresh day in your routine, then you must be able to choose fresh breakfast recipes for yourselves. Breakfast is essential for any day, which has tons and tons of work and you remain the breakfast you eat in your day. Following are some of the fresh ketogenic breakfasts that can be productive for your day

1. French toast

This breakfast is widely shared and eaten throughout the world. French toast has all the necessary ingredients that boost energy in your bodies and the ingredients are especially ketogenic in their nature. It is easily made and it gives all the proper intake to the body chain of energies. It can be made with amalgamating pieces of bread and have a sharp linger of egg on it. French toasts are recommended by doctors to the patients, who have to fight inflammatory diseases.

2. Apple Pancakes

Apple pancakes are the great treasury for you if you strive for a ketogenic diet. This diet is recommended by the entire in all ifs and buts of life. A beautiful mixing of apples in sweat odors of a cake is essential for its making. With a cup of tea, apple pancakes are the healthiest ketogenic diet of all. Also, these pancakes are very easy to make and they can be given in all ranges of prices to the customers.

For its making, you need a half cup of flour, a half teaspoon of grounded cinnamon, an egg whisked, one-third cup full of milk, two red apples, cooking oil, blueberries and low-fat frozen yogurt. With these ingredients, the apple pancakes can be easily made and there is a lot of delicious taste attached to it.

3. Avocado Breakfast Salad

This breakfast salad can help you regain all your lost energies in you when you are sleeping. It is the Mexican salad that can help you give important details to your intake at all the possible levels of your body. Its ingredients are two tortillas, half a spoon of firm tofu, one avocado, a handful of almonds, one spoon of chili sauce, half a red onion and half a lemon. It makes is very simple as well and every layman, who wants a fast and healthy diet can use this salad for its own making.

4. Mix Sprout Salad

If you want to start your day with a tasteful ketogenic diet then mix sprout is the best salad for you. It has the proteins, vitamins, minerals and energy ounces that can be very instrumental for you. Its ingredients include fifty grams of sprouts, one cucumber, one spring onion, a handful of parsley, fresh juice of a lemon, Celtic sea salt, and black pepper.

The making of it is also very fundamental for you and it gives you the best amount of energy you can possibly have.

5.   Kale Chickpea Mash

This dish, with its name, sounds very tasty for you and it provides all the necessary benefits for your side. The ingredients for its make contain three tablespoons of garlic, one shallot, a bunch of kale, four hundred grams of chickpeas, two tablespoons of coconut oil and Celtic tea taste for more relish. The making of this recipe is also very easy. You just need to chop out the salad in an equal manner and add some minced garlic in olive oil. Then you have to wait till it turns golden brown and then you can add some onion and garlic. Add some chickpeas and start to cook them. Put the remaining ingredients in it and pour it in it and after proper mixing, your dish is now ready to be served.

6. Quinoa and Apple Breakfast

This breakfast food has a great combination for it. It has the finest ingredients involved in it. The ingredients are a half cup of quinoa, one apple, half a lemon, and cinnamon. These ingredients will produce the finest ketogenic breakfast for you that will have all the healthy proteins, enzymes and vitamins for you. In order to create it, you have to cook the quinoa first, you have to add some water, you have to boil the water for fifteen minutes, grate the apple and cook for thirty seconds, sprinkle some cinnamon and add raisins for a flowery taste.

7. Cold Oats

The col oat dish is an amazing breakfast ketogenic food for you that can give you early breakfasts for good metabolism. The ingredients of this meal contain half a cup of oats, half a skimmed of meat, half a cup of yogurt, half a teaspoon of cinnamon, a banana sliced, a cup of berries and a table teaspoon of berries. The steps are very easy to understand. First and foremost is the mixing of oats, seal the mixing in a jar and put it in the refrigerator, add banana slices and berries with cinnamon in the morning and after it bake it for good use.

8.   Scrambled Tofu

Let us assume that you are a corporate owner and you have to go early on your job for a good lifestyle and attention, the best breakfast that you can have is scrambled tofu. The ingredients are one union, three cloves, three tomatoes, some firm tofu, half a teaspoon of cumin, half a teaspoon of paprika, half a teaspoon of turmeric, half a cup of yeast, baby spinach and salt for taste. These ingredients are great for a tonic taste for the diet and they can enough relish to the taste as well. The steps are very crucial as well. These are dicing of the onion, mincing of the garlic, the addition of some onions in a pan, the addition of some tofu and some tomatoes, the addition of cumin, paprika, and water, stirring of water and cook, the addition of spinach and flowering of the taste as well.

9. Theplas

In the southern states of Punjab of the subcontinent, Pakistan, and India, theplas is a Gujarati diet that is very ketogenic in its formation. It has ingredients of coriander, garlic, onion, spinach, salt, soya flavor, turmeric, sesame seeds, ragi flour, and capsicum. These ingredients all fill up to be a proper breakfast diet for you and you have to do the careful making of it. The steps are the addition of some oil in a pan and the heating of it for two minutes, the addition of some onion and stirring in your golden oven, the addition of capsicum, paneer, coriander, and salt and cooking for it for two minutes. Removing of the flame and letting it cool for minutes. Further comes the division of dough, cooking helps in oil. Place stuffing on top and serve it fresh.

10. Maple Millet Porridge

A diet filled with protein and amino acids for you. These ingredients are one cup of millet, ten cups of water, a pinch of salt, one tablespoon of cinnamon and a quarter of maple syrup, which can be very productive for the human body. The steps include the taking of a large pot and boiling water for a minute, the addition of some salt and millet, the covering of lid and reduction of heat while doing it, the addition of cinnamon and almond water, the adjusting of the thickness of the food and then dishing is ready.

Therefore, these are breakfast dishes that are ketogenic in nature. They must be eaten and highly encouraged in the daily life routine. They are very easy to eat and very nice to cook. You can have all the joys and jollies while you eat them and do not others fool you about it.

Lunch Recipes

We have carefully examined the breakfast diets for you and now, it is the time to discuss the lunch recipes for you. Ideally, for a ketogenic lunch recipe, we have the fruits and other non-dairy products that can be attributed to lunch recipes. However, there are many other lunch recipes that can be used for lunch diets. The lunch recipes are as follows:

1.   Summer Salad with citrus dressing

Salads make a fantastic lunch and if you dress them with juices and sprinkle salts on them then they can make good use of the health as well. You have to do all the cutting and dressing and must try your best in getting the greenish salads for your own benefit. You can only reap benefits for yourself if you are able to amalgamate tomatoes, carrots, green-leaved, cabbage and lemons in the salad. For a salty taste, you can sprinkle some salads on the salad for your own relish. This meal is very conducive for your health and can be used in many situations while you want a lunch meal for you. You have to very keen while looking at this situation and you will get all the amazing results to your body if you have a salad for yourself.

2.   Cheesy Kale Chips and Sliced Fruit

These kips contain all the necessary amount of minerals, amino acids, proteins, and enzymes the human body needs. They are very easy to be made and you can gain a lot of energy while you are eating them. You can have all the amount of relish while you eat them and you are able to get away from the stubbornness that your body takes. Plus, these chips also contain a sliced portion of fruits for you. Fruits, coupled with salad can be very productive for your health. In this way, you can achieve all the accumulation of enjoyment that you can get.

3.   Green Apple Slices with Raw almond butter

An almond contains infinite pieces of energy for your body and you can get all amount of relish while eating them. While green apple slices are available in all ranges and prices for you, the almonds that you will add in them will create another tone for you. These green apples are sliced, which means that it can create a taste of juice for you. With almond butter, you have an intake of amino acids for you and thus, this diet can serve as a total package. All you need to do is to follow the regulations while creating it and you can end being very popular in your locality.

4.   Apple Cabbage Salad with Beetroot

A crunchy salad for you, which is very ketogenic in its nature and can be helpful throughout the year; it has an easy process of its making. You need an apple, a cabbage, tomatoes and green leaves for. The beetroot is able to condense the fat intake in proper chemicals that can be helpful for you. You can stay alert in your busy routine throughout the year and you can get all the amount of relishes for yourself. You are able to give proper satisfaction to your clients any way in your duty. This diet can reduce the amount of acidity with full intellect and zeal. You are able to strive for excellence and betterment in all ways possible. You feel great and have a decent amount of excellency in your lifestyle.

5.   Zucchini Sushi

If you are a sushi lover and want to maintain a ketogenic state of your body then zucchini sushi is the real deal for you. You can get all the possibilities of relishes while making it and your body will be able to perform well. You can also do the filling for yourself and can in time, be very healthy while doing it. The dip of it is super flavorful and you can get the taste of it in all possible ways. The ingredients for this diet are four zucchinis, a quarter cup of parsley,

I artichoke hearts, two cloves of garlic, one lemon, which is fresh juices and one can of white beans. You can slice the juicy zucchini in all the possible directions and mix the ingredients for a healthy amount of processing in it. You can also spread the zucchini for all the possible taste and can get satisfaction for it.

6. Courgetti and Quinoa Salad

The ingredients of this salad are very healthy for our body. These are washed and sliced courgettes. These are one cup quinoa, one cup cumin, one tin chickpeas, which are rinsed well and drained, one garlic clove, which is crushed with sea salt, three tablespoons of extra virgin oil, two tablespoons are lemon juice, two spring onions that are chopped properly and small handful flat-leaf parsley leaves. The method to create such a diet is also very impressive. Add the quinoa to a pot, add a cup of water, bring to the boil over medium heat and then simmer it for ten minutes until all the water is properly absorbed. Replace the lid and make all the ingredients mix with it properly. After doing it, heat the olive oil in a large pan. Addition of courgettes is the next step. Cook with the stirring until bright green and tender spoon. Spoon it into a bowl, season and set aside. Replace the pan over medium heat; add the cumin and heat, stirring until fragrant. In the last step, add the spiced oil to the courgettes.

In the last add the chickpeas, quinoa, garlic, extra virgin oil, lemon juice, spring onions, and parsley and toss them well.

7.   Cauliflower Gnocchi

This diet is very vegan and great in its formation. The ingredients include one head of cauliflower, one cloves of garlic, one cup of flour, one tablespoon of olive, one tin of white tomatoes, five courgettes of thickly sliced salads, half onions that are finely sliced, one tablespoon of olive and coconut, two cloves of garlic, six large of mushrooms and three hundred milliliter of vegetable stock. You need to place the cauliflower and garlic in a food blender first. Then you must do a little smoothing. You must add a little salt odor to it as well. So, in this way, a protein-enriched ketogenic diet is at your service and it will yield many proper results as well.

8. Kaule and cucumber kimchi

This green ketogenic diet is very beneficial and healthy for you. It gives you a great amount of protein, amino acids and triggers pro-active digestion in your body. Its ingredients are white cabbage, kale, which is chopped, sea salt, dried chili flakes, smoked paprika, garlic, ginger and a heavy dose of mineral water. You have to stir the ingredients properly. The squeezing of vegetables is very important and you can squeeze the vegetables for five minutes. With this method, natural water can easily come out of the vegetables and will provide a great amount of taste. The tips are as under: leave it on a kitchen counter, away from direct sunlight, next is the fermentation of the mixture for three weeks and then you are allowed to taste it. There are many tips while you prepare this dish. As this is the dish that required jars for your health, therefore; you can sterilize glass jars. For a hot mixture, the jar needs to be hot. This tip will impact the taste of the dish and will give you a crunchy taste in no time.

9. Cauliflower Tabbouleh Salad

This dish is very ketogenic for your health. The ingredients are one raw head of cauliflower, onion that should be chopped, flat-leaf parsley that must be 125 milliliters, 125 milliliters of mint, same amount of dint, cucumber, which must be finely diced, tomatoes should be there, and one small juice of lemon will add more taste, beef bangers, and fresh herb. The method is very crucial for you to understand. For having a tabbouleh salad, the cauliflower must be dried and washed properly. Cut the fish into chunks and add it into the food processor. The process is fine but it needs to be purified by all means necessary. For having a sausages flow, heat the pan over a pace of medium heat. Add a bit of olive oil for the taste and then dry the sausages for a proper taste. For fresh herbs, you need to add a group of dollops for a fresh and genuine taste.

10. Grilled Courgette Salad

The best ketogenic dish that you can taste for a good relish and a healthy body is grilled courgette salad. It has a spicy list of ingredients that can be very helpful for human metabolism. The ingredients include six courgettes, eighty gram of watercress, sea salt, chili meant dressing, one red chili, and salt. For a better mechanism, the courgettes and watercress can be of high use. You have to slice the courgettes lengthwise, you must give a sprinkle of salts on the salads; do the dressing of salts, wash the lemon, mint leaves, and chili while having a salad make, place the watercress in the serving dish and create more flavor in it by having additional tastes for it. Once you have done all it then you can do the dressing part effectively.

11.   Roasted Vegetable Oil and Coconut Milk soup

This vegetable ketogenic diet is very vane for you. Having ketogenic diets in it gives this dish a very proper and genuine taste. The ingredients of this diet include two shopped vegetables, olive oil, which is used to roast vegetables, salt, and black pepper to taste, one tablespoon of butter, one freshly grated ginger and salt and pepper for a taste. First and foremost, you need to heat it over 180 degrees Celsius; you have to arrange the chopped vegetables in a regular manner, you can add the butter and saute the garlic and ginger, you may also add the coconut milk and simmer it for thirty minutes, once this is done you can transfer coconut milk to a bowl and add vegetables to it. These tactics will help to ensure the taste you desire in the diet.

12. Crunchy quinoa salad

This crunchy quinoa salad is very good and delicious for your healthy state of mind. Without its use, the autophagy of the body can be easily processed. The ingredients of the salad contain raw quinoa, raw butternut, raw cauliflower, olive oil, cucumber, raw carrot, kale, mint, Danish feta, pumpkin seeds, salt and pepper, lemon vinaigrette, wholegrain mustard, and parsley. These dishes can be very helpful for you as they give enough taste and autophagy in the body. All such tactics require a sheer sense of mixing and food dynamics and one should always abide by the notion of cleanliness first. In a frying pan, you need to heat a little olive oil. Pan Fry cauliflower until they are colored. You need to place all vinaigrette ingredients into a jug blender and blend them together. Also, mix them with lemon vinaigrette and toss them upside down.

Thus, these lunch recipes will serve the taste of ketogenic lunch recipes for you and you will get all the relish and quality of freshness while you are eating it.

Dinner Recipes

We all want a satisfying and delicious dinner that can end our routines and also the dinner that gives us less fat while we are sleeping. For such dinners, we have to search and must come up with autophagy in them. These are the dinners which will make your bodies look lean and aesthetic. These recipes along with their mechanisms are as follows:

1. Brilliant Beet Lattles

Beet lattles can be very helpful for your bodies as they provide enormous impacts of energies. If you add a pouring of almond milk in the lattle, it will be very helpful for you. You have to be quite specific in this regard. The beet lattle is very colorful and it is also creamy. The creation of this epic diet is very easy. You need to follow all the mechanism related to it. The mechanism involves tenacious workings. It starts with the pouring of two almond kinds of milk into the blender; for this purpose, you have to use strained milk. Then you add some preferred sweetener to it. The sweetener can be dates or birch xylitol to it. After the addition of two teaspoons of beet powder, vanillas extract and ginger to it. Then is the use of high-speed blender that gives a friction heat of blades to the public. Secure the lid of the blender and then start to mix it up. However, if you are using a conventional machine then you have to give more mixing to the ingredients.

This single beet powder can be of very uses. The first use is in an almond milk latte, boost the content and nutrient content of smoothies, give more taste to raw alkalis, also in smoothies and workload, and you may add color to the pancakes as well if you are using the beetles. Also, there is a pasta flavor to it. There can be a gorgeous color to the salads and also, there can be a natural food coloring to the toy dough as well.

Beet lattle has a lot of health benefits as well. It is loaded with vitamins, minerals, antioxidants, dietary fiber, and nutrients. This compound, which is ketogenic in its nature can give stronger blood regulations, can give cellular healing, can give oxygen uptake, improves stamina and tries to give endurance for any mechanical workouts.

2. Gluten-Free Vegan Berry Pie

This pie is a great deal for tonight. As it has all the important requirements that a body needs to get before sleep. It has minerals, proteins and juicy vitamins, which can yield the proper amount of energy for your body. It has a great way of formation. Its mechanism includes the chilling of work bowl in your freezer, wrap your flour packet in a plastic bag, storing it in the freezer, the keeping of fats and at the end, sweeten your fruit for your own good. While sweetening the pie, there are certain modes of it. You have to follow the processing of blueberries, the intake of Marionberries, the use of cherries and the chemical of rhubarb. These experiments help you to give a good dinner ketogenic food that is great for your body. Also, it eliminates any rusted pieces of fat that are present in the body.

3.   Spicy Cashew Tip

A beautiful, rich and creamy texture is all that you will find in the diet and form of spicy cashew tip. It is very fantastic when it comes to serving it at dinner. It is revered by all the families here and there and it gives a great tone of affection when it is served on the table.

You can also do the creamy salad dressing on your foods through the spicy cashew tip. There are many bursting flavors at the core of this diet and it helps to regain a lot of taste in your body while you eat them. The dish is inspired by the Indian Recipes like the potato and cauliflower curry, the spicy aloo gobi, okra masala, and banana cardamom lassi. These are the diets and recipes that can be used in many ways to keep your sleep ketogenic. The autophagy is therefore reserved in these products and you can come up with many other credentials as well.

These are the dinner recipes that give a ketogenic taste to your body. You must try your best in eating and preserving them.

Chapter 6 - Autophagy for muscle mass

Intermittent fasting

The concept of intermittent fasting means that you have to fast at regular intervals of the daily routine. The autophagy works tremendously under such circumstances and with the passage of time, the working length can be achieved mordaciously. However, there are certain techniques that need to be compensated while you are doing intermittent fasting. They are as follows:

1. The ketosis states

It is a state of intermittent fasting in which the body is able to lower down its metabolic rate and all the saturated fats, located in various parts of the body are easily eliminated. You tend to start this while you are at the 12th hour of your body level and this state forces you to be away from all those bad things that are quite hectic for your body. You become all composed and compassionate in your self while you are at this diet and thus, you are all good to come and proceed in the coming.

2. The recycling of cells

During the second state of the body, the body is able to do the recycling of cells. The cell line is so lenient and efficient in this scenario that you become very effective in this regard. The recycling of cells is an autophagy process and helps to improve the circulation of blood in your holistically. Therefore, the use of autophagy is tremendously very effective for your body to work on and with this, you are able to make a better transition in your body by all means necessary.

3. The 54 hours shift

By this state, the insulin level has dropped by 54 percent and you are feeling very relaxed and better in your style. This the hours' shift that helps you to lessen any composed fat on your waistline and with the passage of time, you are able to be very strong and sustainable in your requirement. Therefore, these three stages are a must to learn states of intermittent fasting and anyone, who desires to have an autophagy run in it, the 54 hours shift is the best shift for it.

Incorporating intermittent fasting

In order to incorporate intermittent fasting in you. You have to adopt the following things in yourself.

1. Be patient and composed

This means that any diet that has a good number of intakes in it and can deliver a better potential in you with the passage of time, it is essential and effective for you. The idea in this scenario is that you have to look for diet and body ideas that can be helpful for you in a coherent level and could engage the best out of you. This might be a little problematic at first but with the passage of time, you will be able to harness it.

2. Always look for a green diet

The green diet will help you to pay a better benefit to your body. You will be able to see how the body language is able to incorporate better standings in you and with the passage of time, you are able to furnish yourself to the next level. Therefore, it is important for you to understand that looking for a green diet for you is the best thing ever happen to you and you must incorporate it in the coming time.

Into your workout plan

The keto diet and the process of autophagy should be incorporated in your work out plan. You must be able to see how the work out is able to make you stand out in front of any issue. You must incorporate physical exercises that could be very effective for your brain and could make you very established in physique as well. Therefore, the incorporation of a workout plan is necessary for you to understand how the body is being moved with possible direction and how autophagy can help to relate in this manner.

Chapter 7 Foods that stimulate autophagy

Following are some of the foods that stimulate autophagy

Ginger

Ginger is a food that stimulates autophagy ghastly and makes things come close in an effective manner.

Green Tea

Green tea is the best drinking lot that can help you to be lean and adopt autophagy in you. It has some herbs and essential ingredients that are designed to give better illustrations to the people. The green tea is easy to mix and can be capitalized easily in the coming time. The green tea requires no such working in the products and can be available in every possible direction

Reishi Mushrooms

Reishi mushrooms can be easily accepted in the world timings and these mushrooms could be made out of nowhere. The mushrooms make the body language more lenient in its desire and with the passage of time, the people are able to learn a lot from its core and construct. The constructs of the mushrooms need to be identified with the passage of time and they are best to carry out an autophagy product.

Turmeric/curcumin

Turmeric is a regimental disease that could be very healthy and compatible with autophagy. It does not require a lot of working for its process and it could easily up bring the concept of better regulations in the time. Therefore, the turmeric and curcumin are the best details looking forward to the people in the society.

Chapter 8 - Stimulating Autophagy by mimicking food

Example of a Fasting-Mimicking diet protocol

Some meat plans are offered in this scenario to make the reader know about the formation of a fast mimicking diet

Basics of the fasting-mimicking diet and its importance in lifestyle

First, let us discuss what is meant by a lifestyle? The lifestyle of an individual is based on his daily routine, his calorie intake, his daily processions, and the repute; he carries along with him while pursuing the daily lifestyle. The lifestyle of a starlet can be very famous. He will ride new vehicles; he will look healthy and try his best to do the best in his movies. He will professionalize his life by working hard and he will adopt a healthy regime in his routine to be successful. Therefore, the daily choices, in terms of food, clothing and routine procession, a lifestyle can be defined.

Now why the alkaline lifestyle is so popular? What basic ingredients, it holds in it that makes it famous. The result of having a fast mimicking diet is very successful in its reflection and the confidence that any individual can harness through it is the real reason why the intake of a fast mimicking diet can be very effective. People deem it famous because they become famous or at-least become renowned to the fact that they are in the limelight. The idea of popularity can be assessed through this notion that eating a fast mimicking diet can make you fit and being fit, can be the source of a healthy lifestyle. While having a lifestyle, you can do a lot of works, a lot of practice and can execute many frameworks through effective planning. This argument can be further prolonged to many levels of analysis.

The first level of analysis is the individualistic level. On an individualistic level, individuals get revered to be the lean and muscular figures that have the potential to succeed in life. They can do a lot of things like move composedly in their professional careers, they can be the focus on their diets and prevent their bodies from being affected by many health diseases like TB, heart cancer, kidney stone and even fracture of bones. They can go to popular lifestyles like the fashion industry and even apply for acting careers. Therefore, on an individualistic level, one can easily transform the credentials of his self into a famous personality. All he needs to do is to have a fast mimicking diet in his routine.

On a social level, a society steams into the portions of activeness and recognition through a fast mimicking diet. A society is able to get all the intention and popularity if it follows a fast mimicking diet because the functions of society and the correlation of social institutions can be effective in their progress and allowing the intake of a fast mimicking diet will always open a plethora of opportunities for the society to flourish in the status-quo. Also, the norms and values are equally translated into the successful sustenance of any society and the claws of societal decadence are easily averted. So, on a societal level, there are many features of having a fast mimicking diet that can be very helpful for a society to boost its formation in the contemporary. All the societies, whether western or eastern, must be allowed to have a taste of this fast mimicking diet and this diet could be effective for the nourishment of their lifestyles.

The state-level can also be analyzed while discussing the popularity of a fast mimicking diet. The state is an engine for any country's progress and without its efficient working and statehood; a nation cannot become successful in geopolitics and geo-economics. Leaders need to adopt a fast mimicking diet system that can be healthy for their country's lead and they can steer the nation's ship with productive body metabolisms. For instance, the food regimen of China's President, Mr. Xi Jinping is of significance. The guy does not claim to have a fast mimicking diet but still, his bodily gestures coupled with prudent state policies make him be a decisive state man. Also, there are many leaders that abhor such a food style and hence, the leaders of a state, if they are using an alkaline, they become popular while exhibiting an alkaline lifestyle.

Thus, the modes of working, daily routines and lifestyle are all affected by the proper intake of a fast mimicking diet. Hence, on a social, individualistic and state level, the use of a fast mimicking diet can trigger many bodily changes in a human body and this is all the cause of the popularity of a fast mimicking diet.

Day one

For day one, the following description must be followed to get a comprehensive change to a body.

1.   Breakfast

Breakfast will be strawberry cocoa chia quinoa. The ingredients for this breakfast are one cup cooked quinoa, two dates, five chia seeds, almond pieces, one-half cup of almond, coconut or hemp milk, coconut shredded flakes, four sliced strawberries and a half cup of almond. The direction will be impact-full if you follow it with strict rules. The night before you cook quinoa, you have to be very diligent. Cook quinoa and strawberry chia before cooking the quinoa and mix the strawberries, almond milk and two dates in a blender. Puree them until they are smoothed. Pour the mixture of the jar and add chia seeds to it. You have to do the mixing until all the seeds are covered with milk. Cover it with the lid and refrigerate overnight. In the morning, when you wake up you must place chia seeds in a bowl and add the quinoa in a homogeneous manner. Enjoy the shredded coconut and serve it to your meal.

2. Lunch

Lunch will be the sweet and savory salad. The ingredients are one large head of butter lettuce, cucumber sliced, cup apple vinegar, one pomegranate, extra virgin oil, one avocado cubed, one garlic clove and quarter cup shelled pistachios. The directions for this recipe are: You have to hand and tear the lettuce in a salad bowl and then add the rest of the ingredients.

Day two

The following description should be kept in mind while following the plan on day two.

1. Breakfast

Breakfast will be a nondairy apple parfait. Ingredients contain half cup-soaked cashews, one cup chopped apple, half cup unsweetened almond or coconut milk and vanilla. Directions contain the combinations of cashews, almond milk, and vanilla in a blender and their blending until you smooth them. The layering of the ingredients in a small cup is the next step. Heaping of the spoon of cashew cream and dressing the top with oats must be there to see the finish the diet.

2.   Lunch

Lunch will be a savory avocado wrap. The ingredients for this recipe are one butter lettuce, one tablespoon of cilantro, half of the avocado, quarter red onion, one tablespoon of chopped basil, a small handful of spinach and sea salt and pepper. Direction includes the spreading the avocado onto a leaf and sprinkle the dish with salt, basil, cilantro, red onion, and spinach. This final dressing will be pertinent to ensure the taste of the dish in all the possible directions.

Day three

In the third day, following recipes need to be followed:

1. Breakfast

Breakfast will be an almond butter crunch berry smoothie. The ingredients will be two cups fresh spinach, one banana, two cup almond milk, four raw almond butter, one cup of any of strawberries, grapes and mixed berries. One tablespoon of chia. Directions include the blending of spinach and almond first milk. Add remaining ingredients except for chia and blend it in. Add more chia once the mixture is all smooth. If you do not possess a valuable speed blender then you must mix more chai in the ingredients. Just sit for a moment and enjoy it with full esteem.

2. Lunch

Lunch will be kale pesto pasta in this scenario. Its ingredients include one bunch kale, sea salt, and pepper, two cups fresh basil, one zucchini, which is noodled, a quarter cup of extra virgin oil, half cup walnuts, garnish with sliced asparagus, spinach leaves, and tomato, two limes and fresh sprinklers of salt. Directions are very pertinent to follow when there are such recipes to eat. In the night, you need to soak walnuts to give absorption. Put all ingredients in the blender or food processor, and blend it until you get cream of consistency. In the end, add some zucchini noodles.

Day four

The following description must be added to witness the intake on day four.

1. Breakfast

Breakfast will be apple and almond butter oats. The ingredients will be two cups of gluten-free oats, one cup grated green apple, half cup of coconut oil, one teaspoon of cinnamon and one by three raw almond butter. The directions include the addition of oats, coconut milk, and almond butter into a bowl and mix well. After it, stir the mixture in the mixture in the grated apple, cover the bowl with a lid or plastic wrap and place it in the refrigerator. Refrigerate overnight. If the oats get too thick, add some coconut milk to like them. In the end, garnish the mixture with cinnamon powder.

2. Lunch

Lunch will be Green Goddess bowl with avocado cumin dressing. Ingredients are divided into different dressings. The first dressing is for avocado cumin dressing. Ingredients include the presence of one avocado, one cumin powder, two limes, one cup filtered water, quarter tablespoon sea salt, extra virgin oil, dash cayenne pepper, a quarter of smoked paprika. The other dressing is the ingredients are for Tahini Lemon Dressing. The ingredients include a quarter cup of tahini, half cup of filtered water, half lemon, which is freshly squeezed, one clove minced garlic, quarter sea salt, dash cayenne pepper, smoked paprika, black pepper to taste and minced garlic. The other layer is for salad. Ingredients include three cups kale, half cup key noodles, half cup broccoli florets, cherry tomatoes, half zucchini, and hemp seeds. The directions of this lunch recipe are lightly steamed kale and broccoli for four minutes, mix zucchini noodles, kelp noodles, toss with a generous serving of smoked avocado and have a cumin dressing. Add cherry tomatoes in it and toss them again. Next, you need to plate the steamed kale and broccoli and try to drizzle them with lemon tahini dressing. Top kale and broccoli with the dressed noodles and tomatoes. In the end, sprinkle the whole dish and hemp them with seeds.

Day five

The description is composed of the following diets

1. Breakfast

For breakfast, we have the berry good spinach power smoothie. The ingredients for this recipe are two cups of fresh spinach, one coconut oil, two cups of unsweetened almond milk, one tablespoon of cinnamon, one cup from mixed berries, one raw almond butter and one frozen banana. The direction is that you need to blend spinach and almond milk first then you can add the remaining ingredients to the mixture.

2. Lunch

Lunch, in this scenario, will be a quinoa burrito bowl. The ingredients for this recipe include the cup of quinoa, four garlic cloves, two hundred and fifteen cans of black beans, one heaping cumin, four green onions sliced, two avocados sliced and two limes fresh juiced. The direction in this recipe will be the cooking of quinoa to get a good shape of quinoa. Then you have to warm the beans for your intake. When quinoa is done cooking then you have to divide the mixture in various serving bowls.

You need to top with beans, avocado, and cilantro.

Day six

This day will have the following recipes to start with.

1. Breakfast

Breakfast will be quinoa morning porridge. The ingredients will contain a half cup of rinsed quinoa, chia seeds, can of coconut milk, hemp seeds, and cinnamon. The direction will be the combination of all the ingredients except the hemp seeds and simmer them for 10-15 minutes until liquid is absorbed. Sprinkle them with hemp seeds.

2. Lunch

Lunch will be thai quinoa salad. The ingredients for dressing will be chopped seeds, cup tahini, lemon-fresh juiced, one pitted date, one teaspoon of apple cider vinegar, one salt, one tamari, and gluten-free and toasted sesame oil. Ingredients for salad will be one cup of quinoa steamed, one tomato sliced, one large handful of arugula and a quarter of red onion sliced. Directions include the blending of all the following, filtered water first and then the rest of all the ingredients. Then you can blend them. After it, you have to steam one cup of quinoa in a steamer or rice cooker and then you can set aside things. Combination of all the quinoa, arugula, sliced tomatoes, diced red onion, onto a serving plate and bowl and then add thai dressing and hand mix with a spoon and serve.

Day seven

The description is as follows for this day.

1. Breakfast

Breakfast will be an alkaline warrior chia breakfast. The ingredients are one cup of unsweetened almond or coconut milk, one tablespoon of unsweetened shredded coconut flakes, four tablespoons of chia seeds, vanilla, cinnamon, chopped nuts, and hemp seeds. The direction includes a combination of milk and chia seeds in a mason jar. Add vanilla, cinnamon, and chopped nuts. Then you can cover the lid with the mixture until it is combined. Refrigerate the mixture overnight. The next morning shake it or stir it with two or three bowls. Top it with optional fresh fruit, coconut shreds, and more chopped fruits.

2. Lunch

Lunch will be the Asian Sesame dressing and noodles. The ingredients will include two tablespoons of tahini, one tamari, liquid coconut nectar, lemon-fresh squeeze, and ingredients will be one scallion, one tablespoon raw sesame seeds, sliced red bell pepper, and carrot. The direction for the lunch will be the choice of either chopping the noodles or using a zucchini. In a mixing bowl, combine all the dressing ingredients and thoroughly mix the spoon. Make your zucchini noodles with a spiralizer or if using kelp noodles, place in warm water for ten minutes to rinse off the liquid, they are packaged with, allowing them to separate and soften. Add the Asian sesame for your dressing and mix it thoroughly. You will have a great amount of relish and comfort for your digestion.

Follow a similar plan for the remaining twenty-three days. The entire meal plan has to be similar to an equal amount of intake and balance. The dinner can be any from the dinner recipes and try your best in maintaining a lesser intake of dinner.

Day Eight

The description is as follows for this day.

1.   Breakfast

Breakfast will be French toast. The ingredients are bread, egg and heating pan. You need to careful while padding the bread in the jar. The direction includes a combination of milk and chia seeds in a mason jar. Add vanilla, cinnamon and chopped nuts for a good flavor. Then you can cover the lid with the mixture until it is combined. Refrigerate the mixture overnight. The next morning shake it or stir it with two or three bowls. Top it with optional fresh fruit, coconut shreds, and more chopped fruits.

2. Lunch

Lunch will be the summer salad with citrus dressing. Salads make a fantastic lunch and if you dress them with juices and sprinkle salts on them then they can make good use of the health as well. You have to do all the cutting and dressing and must try your best in getting the greenish salads for your own benefit. You can only reap benefits for yourself if you are able to amalgamate tomatoes, carrots, green-left, cabbage and lemons in the salad. For a salty taste, you can sprinkle some salads on the salad for your own relish. This meal is very conducive for your health and can be used in many situations while you want a lunch meal for you. You have to very keen while looking at this situation and you will get all the amazing results to your body if you have a salad for yourself.

Day Nine

The description is as follows for this day.

1.   Breakfast

Apple pancakes are the great treasury for you if you strive for an alkaline diet. This diet is recommended by the entire in all ifs and buts of life. A beautiful mixing of apples in sweat odors of a cake is essential for its making. With a cup of tea, apple pancakes are the healthiest autophagy of all. Also, these pancakes are very easy to make and they can be given in all ranges of prices to the customers. For its making, you need a half cup of flour, a half teaspoon of grounded cinnamon, an egg whisked, one-third cup full of milk, two red apples, cooking oil, blueberries and low-fat frozen yogurt. With these ingredients, the apple pancakes can be easily made and there is a lot of delicious taste attached to it.

2. Lunch

These kips contain all the necessary amounts of minerals, amino acids, proteins, and enzymes the human body needs. They are very easy to be made and you can gain a lot of energy while you are eating them. You can have all the amount of relish while you eat them and you are able to get away from the stubbornness that your body takes. Plus, these chips also contain a sliced portion of fruits for you. Fruits, coupled with salad can be very productive for your health. In this way, you can achieve all the accumulation of enjoyment that you can get.

Day ten

The description is as follows for this day.

1. Breakfast

The breakfast will be the avocado salad. This breakfast salad can help you regain all your lost energies in you when you are sleeping. It is the Mexican salad that can help you give important details to your intake at all the possible levels of your body. Its ingredients are two tortillas, half a spoon of firm tofu, one avocado, a handful of almonds, one spoon of chili sauce, half a red onion and half a lemon. Its make is very simple as well and every layman, who wants a fast and healthy diet, can use this salad for its own making.

2. Lunch

Lunch will be green almond slices with rich grains. An almond contains infinite pieces of energy for your body and you can get all amount of relish while eating them. While green apple slices are available in all ranges and prices for you, the almonds that you will add in them will create another tone for you. These green apples are sliced, which means that it can create a taste of juice for you. With almond butter, you have an intake of amino acids for you and thus, this diet can serve as a total package. All you need to do is to follow the regulations while creating it and you can end being very popular in your locality.

These ten meal day plans will ensure fasting-mimicking in your body in a longer span of time.

Chapter 9 - 10 tips to help with fasting

Following are the fresh ten tips to help with fasting

1. Eat fresh

Whenever you want better food for yourself or would want to come up with fasting then you have to start eating fresh. Eating fresh means that all those herbal diets that are available for you must be taken for food installments.

2. Have a clear-sighted goal for eating

While eating never eat junk or bad food just to see how it is. Avoid it at all possible rates.

3. Keep on moving and never stop it

While fasting, belly fat can become a trouble for it. Belly fat becomes stubborn belly fat because it does not get melted. You are sitting and eating and you are gaining much fat without knowing it. What happens is that while sitting and doing no physical exertion, you are gaining visceral fat and the unnecessary fat keeps on improving at your waist. When you will exercise or at least walk or run, you will get a sweat on your belly. The repeated movements will melt the stubborn fat in no time.

4. Load up more proteins

Once you get old, your body produces insulin. Insulin helps gain fat faster and it provides vast storage for fats in the body. Women, who get older and who do not maintain a diet, they feel fat because their bodies do not have a balanced diet. They do not eat vegetables, beef or any other substance that offers proteins and instead they compile a lot of fat on their waist. Hence, more protein than fat should be eaten to maintain a balanced diet in your body.

5. Pile on Polyunsaturates

Saturated fats give more fats as compare to polyunsaturated fats. According to a Swedish study, when individuals eat food either in the form of saturated oil or unsaturated oil than the former gives more weight to the client as the latter one. The saturated oils give a boost to visceral fats on the body while the polyunsaturated ones give less weight and energy to the fat. This is for both men and women to study the significance of polyunsaturated and they should use them in their cooking.

6. Sleep early

While you are fasting, try your best in sleeping early. This will help you to get to the best fasting regimen easily. The fasting comes with a strong viewpoint of things properly and with the passage of time, the people are able to have a better style of it in their characters for fasting. Fasting comes with all the pieces and products effectively and therefore, sleeping is a process that can make the neutral of the body closely and energetically. Therefore, do your best in sleeping early and never hesitate while you are fasting.

7. Avoid smoking at all cost

Smoking is injurious to health. It's painful as it drains all the useful vitamins from the body and if done vigorously, can cause lung fatigue, heart failure, anxiety and many other bodily diseases. Out of the total population of the world, seventy-five-person daily smoke and thirty-five of them are prone to heart diseases and other body malfunctions. This is a serious issue and many countries have formulated an anti-smoking policy among adolescents just to cater to the outcomes of smoking. However, in order to dilute the harmful effects of smoking, a process has been introduced called smoking cessation. This article shall discuss the meaning of smoking cessation and its benefits.

Smoking cessation is a process in which the tobacco content of the cigarette is removed for healthy purposes. It also involves behavioral counseling and communicating in a productive manner. Other cessation techniques include dilution in selling cigarettes and approaching the victim in a positive manner. There are 5a's in the smoking cessation process that are asked, advise, assess, assist and arrange. In asking, a person is inquired of the reason why he/she is smoking and further motivation is given to rectify the menace. In advice, the victim is encouraged to quit the smoke and start doing a healthy activity in the coming time. Assessment involves the mental study of the victim's body and how he can be shaped back to normal. Assistance is the motivation given to the victim so that he may come back to the normal state at the earliest. At last, the arrangement is the process of organizing sustainable livelihoods for the victim and giving him/her an emotional asylum to carry on life for a better purpose.

Smoking cessation has many benefits as well. During the process of 5a's, the endeavor elevates the political, social and economic condition of the victim and helps him to regain his life's objectives in a resonant manner. Furthermore, he is given the motivation to sustain his life for better purposes. Distance from smoking impedes the addiction in a person's mind and abates any bodily disease in him. Once the disease is finished and exterminated, normal metabolism rises in the human body and he can do any tasks in a courageous manner. Thereby smoking cessation guarantees a healthy life possible at all outcomes and it furnishes a stable mechanism for all the human beings involved in the process.

Moving forward, smoking cessation is vital to form a strong family bond. Often in addition, the victim tends to isolate himself from the family closure. He feels distant from the family's affiliation and has no inner love for the family's responsibilities. Smoking cessation does the miracle for him and nurtures him for the best in the coming time.

8. Never exercise while on a fast

Do not do exercises while you are on fast as the body system will lose its stamina and will make you look very bad in its comprehension.

9. Never argue with anyone

Do not argue with anyone who is not in a good mode of yourself. The very better place for it is that you have to be very complacent with others and try to have a better fast.

10. Always be positive.

Positivity comes with a strong impression of being in a relationship and while on fast do your best in refraining from any agitation.

Chapter 10 - Tips to help you optimize autophagy

For optimization of autophagy you have to be the following

1. Eat medicines that are hydrated
2. Never argue with anyone as it increases blood cholesterol
3. Always look for good modes
4. Avoid fats and lipids
5. Eat a healthy diet
6. Be honored to have a doctor visit your place
7. The idea of rationality
8. Never fell guilty pleasure of eating fast foods
9. Always research on your body and have good relationships with others
10. Have an immense load of food intake in you
11. Never underestimate the power of suggestions

Conclusion

To conclude the book, you have to be very careful about diet intakes that you do throughout your routine. You need to be curious about every calorie that goes in you. You have been provided with all the reasons in this book about the process of autophagy. Autophagy can give you a healthy ph and can avert any harmful stroke of acidity in the body. Acidity can be dangerous in profuse accumulation fats, rise to inflammatory disease, the rupture in many digestion organs and having a rusted metabolism that does not work in the flow. On the contrary, autophagy can give you a fresh intake of all healthy diets that can be very healthy and caring for you. These diets are present in all formats.

They are in breakfast recipes, the dinner recipes, the lunch recipes, the smoothies and the sweat desserts that can up-satisfaction in your mouth. You do not have to be an expert in medicine to know which diet to follow when. You just have to know the diet intake of your own body and see how you are able to cater to the plight of diseases. You must not be able to compound yourself with the attack of acidity but must have the courage to use these diets and recover at the earliest.

These diets have everything in their DNA. They have the minerals, the enzymes, the protein, the amino acids, and whatnot. Green refluxes along with curing liquids are present in these diets and they come in all whims and fancies of the diet expression. There is no rocket science behind their creation and one has to be very intelligent while creating them. You can also follow this book and will get a splendid amount of results in no time. It is available at an affordable price.

Try your best in avoiding any acidic diet at all costs even if it gives you a great amount of relish. The idea is fats and minerals are very delicious but they come with devious outcomes of fat accumulation and strengths.

You need to understand that long aging is only possible if you have a balanced diet intake and this diet can be only of an alkaline.

To make conclusive remarks of the book about the benefits of an alkaline diet, first and foremost is the sheer activeness that a person tends to achieve while he is eating an alkaline diet. He feels healthy and looks healthy and wants to be doing a lot of things while he is having an alkaline diet. He can think properly and can get rid of inflammatory diseases that can cause him suffering. He has a strong discipline that can be navigated in any way possible and thus, he is the next big thing for his users. Also, the longevity of life in this scenario and truly, autophagy can do a lot of wonders for the individual. Therefore, autophagy has a lot to do for fitness and active-ness in the human body.

Furthermore, If you want to look green and fresh on your face, then the autophagy can be very helpful in this regard. Studies show that autophagy is very popular in making a healthy face for you. The number of herbs and breakfast recipes you have for yourself, up-bring a good amount of freshness on your face as well on your skin. Thus, autophagy is very crucial for having great skin and face.

Autophagy protects bone density and muscle mass. The mineral intake that you get after having autophagy can protect your bone density. The bones need certain minerals that are used to cure the excessive number of hurdles one gets while running. The minerals are given by autophagy and you are able to get a stronger bone for life. If you are a bodybuilder and want to reap the benefits of the bone then you have to accumulate more autophagy in you that can be very beneficial for you. The muscle mass can be secured in an acute manner if you tend to get more and more almonds and other alkaline dietaries. You have to be very lenient when you are having the autophagy because the benefit of autophagy like the muscle mass and the bone density will be instrumental for you. Just always look at the bright side of the diet and you will feel very productive while you do it.

In today's world, tensions are like a haunting disease that wants to remain at your back for no reason. Everywhere you go, you get a tertiary level of tension. There is the tension of graduating, the tension of succeeding in life, the tension of getting a job and tension of whatnot. You believe that tension can be very successive for you but in the latter, it turns out to be adverse. Scientists have claimed very medical drugs for its cure but the only reasonable cure for is the use of an alkaline diet. The enzymes that you get through vegetables lower the risk of your hyper blood tension and then you can achieve all the relish of your lifestyle in no time. Also, your blood level starts to resonate with full capacity and you will feel like a superman every place you go, therefore; hypertension and tensed matters get an upper hand of resolution when you get to know the prospect of an alkaline diet.

You are able to get a lot of chronic pains in your body due to many reasons. You get to the bottom of any problem; you solve it and end up having chronic pain in your body. Chronic pain refers to any tertiary amount of pain in your body and you are able to get to the harmfulness of it in no time. Therefore, chronic pain is the most devastating headache that you can get and the only effective cure of it is the alkaline diet. Yes, the autophagy is very important for you to maintain as the blood level minimizes when lemon or other alkaline water is induced in the body. So, this is another benefit of autophagy and it does not matter if you are a walker, a boxer or even a corporate worker, you must have autophagy in you if you wish to give all that you crave.

In the end, we will only assure you good health and being a beginner, you must waste any further time and order this book in a jiffy.

Because health is wealth nobody became rich while being lazy and stubborn. This book is all that you need and you must get at all costs.

RENAL DIET
COOKBOOK

TOSHIMORI YOICHI,

MARK DANIEL COOKSEY

Table of Contents

Introduction

Definition

Individuals images with bargained kidney capacity must stick to a renal or kidney diet to eliminate the measure of waste in their blood. Squanders in the blood originate from nourishment and fluids that are devoured. At the point when kidney capacity is undermined, the kidneys not channel or evacuate squander appropriately. In the event that waste is left in the blood, it can contrarily influence a patient's electrolyte levels. Following a kidney diet may likewise help advance kidney work and moderate the movement of complete kidney disappointment.

A renal eating routine is one that is low in sodium, phosphorous, and protein. A renal eating regimen additionally accentuates the significance of expending top notch protein and typically restricting liquids. A few patients may likewise need to restrain potassium and calcium. Each individual's body is unique, and along these lines, it is vital that every patient works with a renal dietitian work to think of an eating routine that is customized to the patient's needs.

The following are a few substances that are pivotal to screen to advance a renal eating routine:

Components of a renal diet

Sodium

What is Sodium and its job in the body?

Sodium is a mineral found in most characteristic nourishments. The vast majority consider salt and sodium as tradable. Salt, be that as it may, is really a compound of sodium and chloride. Nourishments we eat may contain salt or they may contain sodium in different structures. Handled nourishments frequently contain more significant levels of sodium due to included salt. Sodium is one of the body's three significant electrolytes (potassium and chloride are the other two). Electrolytes control the liquids going all through the body's tissues and cells. Sodium adds to:

Directing circulatory strain and blood volume

Directing nerve capacity and muscle compression

Directing the corrosive base equalization of blood

Adjusting how much liquid the body keeps or dispenses with

For what reason should kidney patients screen sodium admission?

An excessive amount of sodium can be unsafe for individuals with kidney malady in light of the fact that their kidneys can't sufficiently wipe out abundance sodium and liquid from the body. As sodium and liquid develop in the tissues and circulation system, they may cause:

Expanded thirst

Edema: growing in the legs, hands, and face

Hypertension

Cardiovascular breakdown: overabundance liquid in the circulatory system can exhaust your heart, making it developed and powerless

Brevity of breath: liquid can develop in the lungs, making it hard to relax

In what capacity would patients be able to screen their sodium consumption?

Continuously read nourishment marks. Sodium substance is constantly recorded.

Give close consideration to serving sizes.

Utilize crisp, instead of bundled meats.

Pick crisp leafy foods or no-salt-included canned and solidified produce.

Stay away from handled nourishments.

Look at brands and use things that are most minimal in sodium.

Use flavors that don't list "salt" in their title (pick garlic powder rather than garlic salt.)

Cook at home and don't include salt.

Cutoff all out sodium substance to 400 mg for each supper and 150 mg for each tidbit.

Printable Low Sodium Diet Guidelines

Potassium

What is Potassium and its job in the body?

Potassium is a mineral found in a significant number of the nourishments we eat and is likewise found normally in the body. Potassium assumes a job in keeping the heartbeat standard and the muscles working accurately. Potassium is additionally essential for keeping up liquid and electrolyte balance in the circulatory system. The kidneys help to keep the perfect measure of potassium in your body and they oust abundance sums into the pee.

For what reason should kidney patients screen their potassium admission?

At the point when the kidneys come up short, they can never again evacuate abundance potassium, so potassium levels develop in the body. High potassium in the blood is called hyperkalemia which can cause:

Muscle shortcoming

A sporadic heart beat

Slow heartbeat

Respiratory failures

Demise

In what capacity would patients be able to screen their potassium consumption?

At the point when the kidneys never again control potassium, a patient must screen the measure of potassium that enters the body.

High-potassium-food Tips to help keep the degrees of potassium in your blood safe, try to:

Converse with a renal dietitian about making an eating plan.

Breaking point nourishments that are high in potassium.

Breaking point milk and dairy items to 8 oz every day.

Pick crisp foods grown from the ground.

Stay away from salt substitutes and seasonings with potassium.

Peruse marks on bundled nourishments and stay away from potassium chloride.

Give close consideration to serving size.

Keep a nourishment diary.

Protein

Protein isn't an issue for solid kidneys. Typically, protein is ingested and squander items are made, which thus are separated by the nephrons of the kidney. At that point, with the assistance of extra renal proteins, the waste transforms into pee. Conversely, harmed kidneys neglect to expel protein waste and it gathers in the blood. The best possible utilization of protein is precarious for Chronic Kidney Disease patients as the sum contrasts with each phase of ailment. Protein is fundamental for tissue support and other substantial jobs, so it is critical to eat the prescribed sum for the particular phase of malady as per your nephrologist or renal dietician.

Liquids

Liquid control is significant for patients in the later phases of Chronic Kidney Disease since ordinary liquid utilization may cause liquid develop in the body which could wind up hazardous. Individuals on dialysis regularly have diminished pee yield, so expanded liquid in the body can put superfluous weight on the individual's heart and lungs. A patient's liquid stipend is determined on an individual premise, contingent upon pee yield and dialysis settings. It is essential to pursue your nephrologist's/nutritionist's liquid admission rules.

To control liquid admission, patients should:

Not drink more than what your primary care physician orders

Tally all nourishments that will liquefy at room temperature (Jell-O®, popsicles, and so on.)

Be mindful of the measure of liquids utilized in cooking

How is a renal diet different?

At the point when your kidneys are not filling in just as they should, waste and liquid develop in your body. After some time, the waste and additional liquid can reason heart, bone and other medical issues. A kidney-accommodating supper plan restricts the amount of specific minerals and liquid you eat and drink. This can help shield the waste and liquid from structure up and causing issues. How exacting your supper plan ought to be relies upon your phase of kidney ailment. In the beginning periods of kidney malady, you may have almost no cutoff points on what you eat and drink. As your kidney sickness deteriorates, your primary care physician may suggest that you limit:

Potassium

Phosphorus

Liquids

Potassium is a mineral found in practically all nourishments. Your body needs some potassium to make your muscles work, however an excess of potassium can be perilous. At the point when your kidneys are not functioning admirably, your potassium level might be excessively high or excessively low. Having excessively or too little potassium can cause muscle spasms, issues with the manner in which your heart thumps and muscle shortcoming. On the off chance that you have kidney sickness, you may need to constrain how a lot of potassium you take in. Ask your primary care physician or dietitian on the off chance that you have to restrict potassium. Utilize the rundown beneath to realize which nourishments are low or high in potassium. Your dietitian can likewise assist you with figuring out how to securely eat modest quantities of your preferred nourishments that are high in potassium.

Eat this ... (lower-potassium nourishments)

Apples, cranberries, grapes, pineapples and strawberries

Cauliflower, onions, peppers, radishes, summer squash, lettuce

Pita, tortillas and white breads

Meat and chicken, white rice

Instead of ... (higher-potassium nourishments)

Avocados, bananas, melons, oranges, prunes and raisins

Artichokes, winter squash, plantains, spinach, potatoes and tomatoes

Grain items and granola

Beans (prepared, dark, pinto, and so on.), darker or wild rice

Your primary care physician may likewise guide you to take an exceptional drug called a potassium folio to enable your body to dispose of additional potassium.

Get familiar with high potassium and its treatment here

Phosphorus

Phosphorus is a mineral found in practically all nourishments. It works with calcium and nutrient D to keep your bones solid. Solid kidneys keep the perfect measure of phosphorus in your body. At the point when your kidneys are not functioning admirably, phosphorus can develop in your blood. A lot of phosphorus in your blood can prompt powerless bones that break effectively.

Numerous individuals with kidney infection need to restrict phosphorus. Inquire as to whether you have to restrain phosphorus.

Contingent upon your phase of kidney infection, your primary care physician may likewise endorse a medication called a phosphate folio. This shields phosphorus from working up in your blood. A phosphate folio can be useful, yet you will in any case need to observe how a lot of phosphorus you eat. Inquire as to whether a phosphate folio is directly for you. Utilize the rundown beneath to get a few thoughts regarding how to settle on sound decisions on the off chance that you have to restrain phosphorus.

Eat this ... (lower-phosphorous nourishments)

Italian, French or sourdough bread

Corn or rice grains and cream of wheat

Unsalted popcorn

Some light-shaded soft drinks and lemonade

Instead of ... (higher-phosphorous nourishments)

Entire grain bread

Grain oats and oats

Nuts and sunflower seeds

Dull shaded colas

Liquids

You need water to live, yet when you have kidney malady, you may not require to such an extent. This is on the grounds that harmed kidneys don't dispose of additional liquid just as they should. An excessive amount of liquid in your body can be hazardous. It can cause hypertension, expanding and cardiovascular breakdown. Additional liquid can likewise develop around your lungs and make it difficult to relax.

Contingent upon your phase of kidney infection and your treatment, your primary care physician may guide you to constrain liquid. In the event that your primary care physician discloses to you this, you should reduce the amount you drink. You may likewise need to decrease a few nourishments that contain a ton of water. Soups or nourishments that dissolve, similar to ice, dessert and gelatin, have a great deal of water. Numerous products of the soil are high in water, as well. Ask your primary care physician or dietitian in the event that you have to confine liquids.

On the off chance that you do need to restrict liquids, measure your liquids and drink from little cups to assist you with monitoring the amount you've needed to drink. Limit sodium to assist cut with bringing down on thirst. On occasion, you may at present feel parched. To help extinguish your thirst, you may attempt to:

Bite gum

Flush your mouth

Suck on a bit of ice, mints or hard treat (Remember to pick sans sugar sweets in the event that you have diabetes. Squanders in the blood originate from nourishment and fluids that are expended. Individuals with kidney malady must hold fast to a renal eating regimen to eliminate the measure of waste in their blood. Following a renal eating regimen may likewise support kidney capacity and defer complete kidney disappointment. A renal eating regimen is one that is low in sodium, phosphorous and protein. A renal eating regimen focuses on the significance of expending top notch protein and constraining liquids. Some renal weight control plans may likewise call for constrained potassium and calcium. Each individual is extraordinary, and along these lines, a dietician will work with every patient to think of a renal eating routine that is custom-made to their needs.

What is renal diet for?

A renal diet is for the control of successive elements in your body in order to regulate a firm metabolism in yourself.

Controlling Phosphorous

Phosphorus is a mineral that sound kidneys get free of in the pee. In kidneys that are coming up short, phosphorus develops in the blood and may cause numerous issues counting muscle a throbbing painfulness, fragile, effectively broken bones, calcification of the heart, skin, joints, and blood vessels. To hold your phosphorus levels under wraps, think about the accompanying tips:

1. Breaking point high phosphorus nourishments, for example,

• Meats, poultry, dairy and fish (you ought to have 1 serving of 7-8

ounces)

• Milk and other dairy items like cheddar (you ought to have

one 4 oz. serving)

2. Stay away from high phosphorus nourishments, for example,

• Lima Beans, Black Beans, Red Beans, Black-looked at Peas, White

Beans, and Garbanzo Beans

• Dark, entire or grungy grains

  Refrigerator batters like Pillsbury

• Dried vegetables and natural products

• Chocolate

• Dark shaded soft drinks

3. Remember to take your phosphate fasteners with dinners and tidbits.

• Your primary care physician will endorse a prescription called a phosphate fastener which will be some kind of polymer gel or calcium prescription. You have to accept your phosphate folio as endorsed by your primary care physician. Regularly you will take a phosphate folio with each supper and tidbit.

4. Typically you're eating routine is restricted to 1000 mg of phosphorus for each day

Controlling Potassium

Potassium is a component that is essential for the body to keep a typical water balance between the cells and body liquids. All nourishments contain some potassium; however, some contain bigger sums. Ordinary kidney capacity will evacuate potassium through pee. Kidneys that are not working appropriately can't expel the potassium in the pee, so it develops in the blood. This can be exceptionally perilous to your heart. High potassium can cause unpredictable heart thumps and can even reason the heart to stop if the potassium levels get to high. Normally, there are no side effects for somebody with a high potassium level. In the event that you are worried about your potassium level, check with your PCP, and pursue the tips underneath.

• Usually a renal patient's eating routine ought to be constrained to 2000 mg of potassium every day.

• The accompanying nourishments are high in potassium:

Bananas Avocado Oranges

Squeezed orange Prunes Prune Juice

Tomatoes Tomato Juice Tomato Sauce

Melon Tomato Puree Honeydew Melon

Nuts Papaya Chocolate

Red Beans Milk White Beans

Lima Beans Garbanzo Beans Black Beans

Lentils Split peas Baked Beans

Exceptionally Prepared Potatoes:

1. Strip and cut into 1/8 inch pieces.

2. Absorb 1 cup potatoes 5 cups of water for 2 hours.

3. Channel and flush and channel.

4. Cook in a lot of water.

5. Channel and pound, fry or serve plain.

Controlling Your Sodium

Sodium, or sodium chloride, is a component that is utilized by every living animal to control the water content in the body. Generally a sodium confinement comes in the type of "No Added Salt." This is important in light of the fact that a more noteworthy admission of sodium will result in inadequately controlled circulatory strain and over the top thirst which can prompt trouble holding fast to the liquid confinements in your eating regimen.

To confine your sodium, you should:

• Avoid table salt and any seasonings that end with "salt"

• Avoid salt substitutes (they contain potassium)

• Avoid salty meats, for example, bacon, ham, frankfurter, sausages, lunch meats, canned meats, or bologna

• Avoid salty snacks, for example, cheddar twists, salted saltines, nuts, and chips

• Avoid canned soups, solidified meals, and moment noodles

• Avoid packaged sauces, pickles, olives, and MSG

Controlling Your Protein

Protein is essential to help in development and upkeep of body tissue. Protein likewise plays a job in battling contamination, recuperating of wounds, and gives a wellspring of vitality to the body.

• You should make a point to eat 7-8 ounces of protein consistently. Nourishments that are high in protein incorporate hamburger, pork, veal, chicken, turkey, fish, fish, and eggs.

• 1 egg is equivalent to 1 ounce of protein, and three ounces of protein is practically identical to the size of a deck of cards.

Controlling Your Fluid Intake

Individuals on dialysis regularly have diminished pee yield, so expanded liquid in the body can put pointless pressure on the individual's heart and lungs.

• A liquid remittance for singular patients is determined based on 'pee in addition to 500ml.' The 500 ml covers the loss of liquids through the skin and lungs.

• Most patients won't pee as much once they start Hemodialysis.

The individuals who produce a great deal of pee might have the option to drink more than those who don't deliver pee.

• Between every dialysis treatment, patients are relied upon to increase a little weight because of the water content in nourishments (leafy foods).

• The measure of liquid in a run of the mill day's feast (barring liquids, for example, water, tea, and so forth.) is in any event 500 ml and subsequently anticipated day by day weight addition is between 0.4 – 0.5kg.

• To control liquid admission, patients should:

☐ Not drink more than what your primary care physician orders (normally 4 cups of liquid every day)

☐ Count all nourishments that will liquefy at room temperature (Jell-O® , popsicles, and natural product frosts).

Fast food facts for the renal patient

Fast help eateries give us a speedy, simple, modest chomp when we're in a hurry. Americans love inexpensive food and there are such a significant number of things to browse! A ton of chains are presently advertising lower-fat choices and whenever picked admirably, quick nourishments can be solid AND fit into your renal eating routine. On the off chance that you are a customary through the drive-up window or much of the time eat in at drive-through joints, keep these tips as a main priority.

Some Ordering Tips:

• Burgers and sandwiches are high in sodium since they are pre-salted. This might be troublesome for the brisk help eatery to discard the salt. Make certain to ask before you request.

• Remember that fries and heated potatoes are wealthy in potassium. In any case, in the event that you can't envision a burger without the fries, request a little serving and request unsalted, if conceivable.

• Keep as a main priority that catsup, mustard, and pickles are for the most part high in sodium. Keep toppings, uncommon sauces and dressings to a base. Solicitation that these garnishes be served "as an afterthought" so you can control the sum.

• Beverage measures commonly are enormous or "super-size" and can add to liquid over-burden if the whole drink is devoured. Request a little drink and make certain to consider it part of your liquid stipend.

• Balance inexpensive food things with other nourishment decisions. As you request, think about different nourishments you have eaten or will eat during the day.

• Choose cooked, steamed or barbecued things over profound fat seared nourishments. To cut back the excess from seared things, request the customary assortment rather than the extra firm and evacuate the skin before eating. Evacuating the skin likewise brings down the sodium content since most hitters and coatings normally incorporate seasonings wealthy in sodium. The immense assortment of vegetables and natural products can give you nutrients An and C, folic corrosive and fiber. Be cautious however, an excursion to the plate of mixed greens bar can furnish you with more fat and calories than a hamburger and French fries! There are numerous serving of mixed greens bar things that can without much of a stretch fit into your renal eating routine.

Dining for the Renal Patient

Eating out in eateries can be troublesome when you are on dialysis. A few amazing assets are found in the NFK Publication "Feasting Out with Certainty." If you have a most loved eatery, approach the administrator for a duplicate of the menu to take to your unit dietitian and they can assist you with making great decisions.

Italian Food

Italian eateries offer a great deal of things appropriate for the renal eating routine. The stunt here is to request the sauce as an afterthought. The red based sauces have potassium and the white sauces are high in phosphorus. You can differ the sauces and the kinds of pasta to make fascinating dinners. Pesto sauce is garlic, basil and oil and is a decent other option. Some shellfish and mussel sauces are not tomato or on the other hand cream-based and are great decisions for fish sweethearts. Plates of mixed greens and breads are incredible decisions here; simply request no olives and cheddar. Keep in mind to request the dressing as an afterthought.

It is smarter to keep away from the dishes like lasagna, cannelloni, ravioli and comparable things as they contain high sodium, high potassium, and high phosphorus fixings. Generally Italian eateries additionally offer some sort of flame broiled chicken as an option to their pasta dish. Have the chicken, serving of mixed greens and bread for your dinner and take the pasta home and have with your claim bread and plate of mixed greens for lunch the following day.

Asian Restaurants

These are troublesome spots to eat in light of the high sodium substance. Chinese cafés are the most troublesome in light of the enormous number of blended dishes in with soy, hoisin, and prepared sauces. They all contain salt as well as MSG. Thai nourishments by and large have more flavors and less sodium, habitually you can request sauces as an afterthought. Japanese cafés will likewise serve more spiced nourishments and cook less with sodium.

Renal diet on a holiday

You can have a pleasant Christmas season this year on the off chance that you settle on the correct decisions. Numerous conventional top choices contain an excessive amount of potassium for renal patients. This article will appear you how to appreciate the special seasons without feeling severely or trying too hard. Browse the Occasion Food list beneath.

Hors d'oeuvres

Celery and Carrot Sticks with cream cheddar

Bagel Chips-Unsalted

Bread Sticks

Cream Cheese or Sour Cream and Dill Dip

Chicken Wings (No Salt Added)

Mixed drink Meatballs (No Salt Added)

Wafers Unsalted

Deviled Eggs

Characteristic Tortilla Chips-Unsalted

Popcorn

Pretzels-Unsalted

Shrimp

Renal friendly diets

On the off chance that your primary care physician has endorsed liquor, maintain a strategic distance from high potassium beverages, for example, ridiculous mary's, screw drivers and pina coladas.

◆Go simple on salty nourishments. It will help you from getting parched time and again.

◆For the primary course, pick new, natural meats like capon, hamburger or pork. Maintain a strategic distance from ham and selfbasting turkeys due to the unnecessary sodium.

◆Substitute rice or an additional aiding of stuffing for potatoes to decrease the potassium in your dinner.

◆Remember to check Jell-O® or Jell-O® servings of mixed greens as a major aspect of your treats.

◆Use whipped cream rather than frozen yogurt on treats.

◆If you have a huge feast, go simple on what you eat the following day. Take your phosphate covers with or following the supper.

How to be successful on a renal diet

Balance

The Dietary Guidelines for Americans accentuates the significance of eating a assortment of nourishments. This applies to dialysis patients, as well. You can appreciate all nourishments in balance while following a renal eating regimen. One of the rules states: "Be reasonable: Enjoy all nourishments, simply don't try too hard."

We Encourage You To:

• Slow down while eating. It takes 20 minutes to send the sign that you've had enough to eat.

• Stop eating when full. Patients should leave the table inclination that they can eat somewhat more.

• Have one little aiding of that chocolate cake and appreciate each chomp.

• Enjoy that bit of lasagna twice to such an extent. Eat half in the café and take the rest home to appreciate the following day.

The Goal

The objective for our patients ought to be a solid way of life that can be kept up as opposed to a transient eating regimen that will in all probability be deserted and produce mental uneasiness.

Diet - ceaseless kidney malady

You may need to cause changes to your eating regimen when you to have interminable kidney infection (CKD). These progressions may incorporate restricting liquids, eating a low-protein diet, constraining salt, potassium, phosphorous, and different electrolytes, and getting enough calories on the off chance that you are shedding pounds. You may need to change your eating regimen more if your kidney malady deteriorates, or in the event that you need dialysis.

Capacity

The reason for this eating routine is to keep the degrees of electrolytes, minerals, and liquid in your body adjusted when you have CKD or are on dialysis. Individuals on dialysis need this uncommon eating routine to constrain the development of waste items in the body. Restricting liquids between dialysis medicines is significant on the grounds that a great many people on dialysis pee practically nothing. Without pee, liquid will develop in the body and cause an excess of liquid in the heart and lungs.

Dietary Guidelines for Adults Starting on Hemodialysis

Since you are starting hemodialysis, there might be numerous adjustments in your day by day life. Your primary care physician has likely disclosed to you that you may need to roll out certain improvements in your eating regimen.

How well you feel will rely upon:

Eating the correct kind and measures of nourishment.

Having the hemodialysis medications your wellbeing expert requests for you

Taking the meds your wellbeing expert requests for you.

Your eating regimen is a significant piece of your treatment. Your kidneys can't dispose of enough waste items and liquids from your blood and your body presently has unique needs. Along these lines, you should confine liquids and change your admission of specific nourishments in your eating regimen. The kidney dietitian at your dialysis focus will assist you with arranging an eating regimen for your uncommon needs.

Utilize this pamphlet as a guide until your dietitian readies a customized feast plan for you. You should:

Eat all the higher protein nourishments.

Eat less high salt, high potassium, and high phosphorus nourishments.

Figure out how much liquid you can securely drink (counting espresso, tea, water, and any nourishment that is fluid at room temperature).

Salt and Sodium

Utilize less salt and eat less salty nourishments: This may control circulatory strain. It might likewise help lessen liquid weight gains between dialysis sessions since salt builds thirst and makes the body hold (or clutch) liquid.

Use herbs, flavors, and low-salt flavor enhancers instead of salt

Keep away from salt substitutes made with potassium.

Meat/Protein

Individuals on dialysis need to eat more protein. Protein can help keep sound blood protein levels and improve wellbeing. Protein additionally helps keep your muscles solid, assists wounds with mending quicker, reinforces your safe framework, and improves generally wellbeing. Eat a high protein nourishment (meat, fish, poultry, crisp pork, or eggs) at each dinner, or around 8-10 ounces of high protein nourishments consistently.

3 ounces = the size of a deck of cards, a medium pork hack, a ¼ pound burger patty, ½ chicken bosom, a medium fish filet.

1 ounce = 1 egg or ¼-cup egg substitute, ¼-cup fish, ¼-cup ricotta cheddar, 1 cut of low sodium lunchmeat, 1tablespoon nutty spread, ½ ounce of nuts or seeds

Note: Even however nutty spread, nuts, seeds, dried beans, peas, and lentils have protein, these nourishments are commonly constrained in light of the fact that they are high in both potassium and phosphorus.

Grains/Cereals/Bread

Except if you have to confine your calorie admission for weight reduction and additionally oversee starch consumption for glucose control, you may eat, as you want from this nutrition class. Grains, oats, and breads are a decent wellspring of calories. A great many people need 6 - 11 servings from this gathering every day.

Sums equivalent to one serving:

1 cut bread (white, rye, or sourdough)

½ English biscuit

½ bagel

½ cheeseburger bun

½ frank bun

1 6-inch tortilla

½ cup cooked pasta

½ cup cooked white rice

½ cup cooked oat (like cream of wheat)

1 cup cold oat (like corn drops or fresh rice)

4 unsalted saltines

1½ cups unsalted popcorn

10 vanilla wafers

Maintain a strategic distance from "entire grain" and "high fiber" nourishments (like entire wheat bread, wheat oat and dark colored rice) to assist you with constraining your admission of phosphorus. By constraining dairy–based nourishments you secure your bones and veins.

Milk/Yogurt/Cheese

Point of confinement your admission of milk, yogurt, and cheddar to ½-cup milk or ½-cup yogurt or 1-ounce cheddar every day. Most dairy nourishments are high in phosphorus.

The phosphorus substance is the equivalent for a wide range of milk — skim, low fat, and entirety! On the off chance that you do eat any high-phosphorus nourishments, take a phosphate cover with that supper.

Dairy nourishments "low" in phosphorus:

(get some information about the serving size that is directly for you)

Spread and tub margarine

Cream cheddar

Substantial cream

Ricotta cheddar

Brie cheddar

Non-dairy whipped beating

Sherbet

On the off chance that you have or are in danger for coronary illness, a portion of the high fat nourishments recorded above may not be great decisions for you.

Certain brands of non-dairy creams and "milk, (for example, rice milk) are low in phosphorus and potassium. Approach your dietitian for subtleties.

Organic product/Juice

All organic products have some potassium, however certain natural products have more than others and ought to be constrained or completely dodged. Constraining potassium ensures your heart.

Breaking point or evade :

Oranges and squeezed orange

Kiwis

Nectarines

Prunes and prune juice

Raisins and dried organic product

Bananas

Melons (melon and honeydew)

Continuously AVOID star organic product (carambola).

Eat 2-3 servings of low potassium organic products every day.

One serving = ½-cup or 1 little organic product or 4 ounces of juice.

Pick:

Apple (1)

Berries (½ cup)

Fruits (10)

Organic product mixed drink, depleted (½ cup)

Grapes (15)

Peach (1 little crisp or canned, depleted)

Pear, crisp or canned, depleted (1 divide)

Pineapple (½ cup canned, depleted)

Plums (1-2)

Tangerine (1)

Watermelon (1 little wedge)

Beverages:

Apple juice

Cranberry juice mixed drink

Grape juice

Lemonade

Vegetables/Salads

All vegetables have some potassium, yet certain vegetables have more than others and ought to be restricted or completely dodged. Constraining potassium admission ensures your heart.

Eat 2-3 servings of low-potassium vegetables every day. One serving = ½-cup.

Pick:

Broccoli (crude or cooked from solidified)

Cabbage

Carrots

Cauliflower

Celery

Cucumber

Eggplant

Garlic

Green and Wax beans ("string beans")

Lettuce-different types (1 cup)

Onion

Peppers-different types and hues

Radishes

Watercress

Zucchini and Yellow squash

Point of confinement or stay away from:

Potatoes (counting French Fries, potato chips and sweet potatoes)

Tomatoes and tomato sauce

Winter squash

Pumpkin

Asparagus (cooked)

Avocado

Beets

Beet greens

Cooked spinach

Parsnips and rutabaga

Treat

Contingent upon your calorie needs, your dietitian may prescribe unhealthy deserts. Pies, treats, sherbet, and cakes are great decisions (yet limit dairy-based pastries and those made with chocolate, nuts, and bananas). On the off chance that you have diabetes, examine low sugar dessert decisions with your dietitian.

Test Menu

Breakfast

Cranberry Juice, 4 ounces

Eggs (2) or ½-cup egg substitute

Toasted white or entire wheat bread (2 cuts)

Spread or tub margarine or organic product spread

Espresso, 6 ounces

Lunch

Fish plate of mixed greens sandwich made with 3 ounces fish on a hard move with lettuce and mayonnaise.

(Other great decisions for sandwiches incorporate egg and chicken serving of mixed greens, lean meal meat, low salt ham and turkey bosom.)

Coleslaw, ½-cup

Pretzels (low salt)

Canned and depleted peaches, ½-cup

Soda, 8 ounces

(Cola beverages are high in phosphorus. Pick soda or lemon-lime drinks.)

Supper

Burger patty, 4 ounces on a bun with 1-2 teaspoons ketchup

Plate of mixed greens (1 cup): lettuce, cucumber, radishes, peppers, with olive oil and vinegar dressing

Lemonade, 8 ounces

Go for at any rate 2-3 "fish" dinners every week. Many fish are wealthy in heart-sound "omega-3" fats. Fish and salmon (washed or canned without salt) and shellfish are magnificent heart sound protein decisions.

Tidbit/Dessert

Milk, 4 ounces

Cut of crusty fruit-filled treat

This supper plan gives 2150 Calories, 91 grams protein, 2300 mg sodium, 1800 mg potassium, 950 mg phosphorus. 38 liquid ounces.

In what manner will I know whether I am eating right to remain sound?

Eating admirably causes you remain solid. Eating ineffectively can expand your odds of sickness and influence how you feel. Your dietitian will chat with you about how well you are eating and will assist you with changing your eating regimen to your individual needs dependent on your lab report and discussions with you.

A few inquiries you may be posed:

Have you seen an adjustment in the sort or measure of nourishment you eat every day?

Have you had any issues eating your typical or suggested diet?

Have you shed pounds easily?

Have you seen any adjustments in your quality or capacity to deal with yourself?

Your dietitian or medical attendant may take a gander at the fat and muscle stores in your face, hands, arms, shoulders, and legs. Your dialysis care group will search for changes in your blood level of proteins, and particularly one called "egg whites." An adjustment in this protein can imply that you are losing body protein, yet egg whites can likewise be influenced on the off chance that you have a contamination or are putting on an excessive amount of liquid load between medications. The dietitian may prescribe a protein supplement, for example, Nepro™ or LiquaCel™ to expand protein levels. The dietitian may likewise recommend little incessant dinners and bites. Work with your dietitian to improve your blood level of protein. The perfect measure of dialysis is likewise significant for eating great and remaining solid.

Imagine a scenario in which I have elevated cholesterol.

Changing your eating routine may help bring down the cholesterol level in your blood. Your dietitian will converse with you about the sorts of fat and creature nourishments you eat. Expanding admission of low potassium products of the soil, diminishing the measure of seared nourishments, notwithstanding 150 minutes of physical action every week can improve cholesterol levels. Imagine a scenario where I have diabetes.

From the start the kidney and diabetic eating regimen give off an impression of being altogether different, however they are similar from numerous points of view. The two weight control plans suggest eating 3 adjusted suppers, evading a lot of protein, and restricting sodium. A fair supper has in any event 3 of the nutrition classes (protein, grain, vegetables, natural products, and dairy). The kidney diet confines the measure of milk that you drink, yet numerous individuals with diabetes as of now limit milk to 4 ounces every day. Both prescribe ½ plate of vegetables, ¼ plate of starch rich nourishment, ¼ plate of high protein nourishment, and a bit of organic product. The greatest change is that the kidney diet doesn't have as a lot of assortment in the kinds of foods grown from the ground decisions since some have more potassium than others. The diabetic eating routine prescribes 45 to 75 grams of sugar with every feast and dispersing suppers 4 to 5 hours separated. This suggestion is useful for the kidney diet, as well. Both the kidney and diabetic eating routine assistance to keep your heart solid.

Now and again, you may need to make just a couple of changes in your eating routine to meet your requirements as a kidney quiet. For instance, you may need to constrain a portion of the free nourishments you have been utilizing may should be restricted on your kidney diet. Your dietitian will help make a feast arrangement particularly for you.

Is there something else I should know?

The accompanying significant hints can be useful with your eating regimen:

Crisp or plain solidified vegetables contain no additional salt. Channel all the cooking fluid before serving.

Canned organic products generally contain less potassium than crisp natural products. Channel all the fluid before serving.

Rice and almond milk are low in phosphorus and can be utilized instead of milk.

Marks on nourishment bundles will give you data about a portion of the fixings that may not be permitted in your eating regimen. Figure out how to peruse these marks to assist you with restricting sodium and control phosphorous. Maintain a strategic distance from nourishments with fixings that contain "PHOS"

To assist you with maintaining a strategic distance from salt, numerous herbs and flavors can be utilized to make your eating regimen all the more intriguing. Check with your dietitian for a rundown of these.

Nutrition and Kidney Disease

Most patients in the beginning times of kidney malady need to confine the measure of sodium in their eating regimen. A few patients might be advised to restrain protein in their eating routine too. The DASH diet is frequently suggested for patients with kidney malady. Make certain to converse with your social insurance supplier about your particular sustenance needs.

Diets for Kidney Patients

Dealing with your eating routine with kidney sickness

When living with constant kidney sickness, overseeing what you eat and drink can be a test; notwithstanding, your eating regimen can likewise emphatically impact how you feel, and what different medications you may require. An Accredited Practicing Dietitian experienced in kidney sickness, called a Renal Dietitian, is the best individual to counsel about an individualized feast plan. The initial step will be a dietary appraisal to survey your admission of vitality and significant supplements.

Dietary appraisal incorporates an audit of your admission of vitality and significant supplements, for example,

protein

sodium/salt

potassium

phosphate

liquid

fat

Dietary guidance is given on an individual premise, considering what you like to eat, how you are feeling, your age, way of life, weight, muscle size, wellbeing status and blood test outcomes.

Everybody should constrain their salt, sugar and fat admission as a feature of solid living.

As kidney malady advances, your dietary needs are probably going to change. Your kidneys will turn out to be less compelling at evacuating undesirable liquid and dealing with the right degrees of supplements, for example, calcium, phosphate and potassium. The underlying dietary changes prescribed may be little, yet as your kidney malady advances increasingly critical changes might be required. View our scope of diet and sustenance reality sheets here or perceive how to perceive how to decrease your salt admission here.

In the event that you are now on dialysis, see other valuable eating routine and nourishment tips accessible here. Step by step instructions to capitalize on your meeting with a Renal Dietitian

Over various days before your arrangement, record what you eat and take the rundown with you.

Take a rundown of your drugs.

In the event that another person regularly cooks for you, request that they go with you.

Pose inquiries with the goal that you feel sure about what you have to do and why.

Arrange normal follow-up arrangements to screen your advancement.

The Dietitians Association of Australia can give names and contact subtleties of nearby renal dietitians

Keeping up a sound weight

A few people with incessant kidney infection don't want to eat or experience issues eating enough nourishment to remain sound. Unhealthiness can create when nourishment admission is deficient and your body doesn't get the perfect measure of the nutrients, minerals and different supplements. This is increasingly normal in the later phases of incessant kidney malady.

On the off chance that you are getting thinner that isn't arranged, or have any worries about your eating regimen, tell your primary care physician or renal dietitian. Weight increase can likewise cause genuine medical issues. On the off chance that you are overweight it tends to be more diligently to get entrance for dialysis, and you may likewise not be reasonable for a kidney transplant. On the off chance that weight increase is an issue, your renal dietitian can assist you with arranging a fitting eating program. Prior to taking any dietary enhancements or beginning an arrangement to lose or build weight reduction, consistently look for guidance from your primary care physician or renal dietitian. Changes to your nourishment and liquid admission might be not kidding and cause huge harm.

Tips on nutrients and minerals

In case you're not getting every one of the nutrients and minerals you need from the nourishments you eat, at that point nutrient and mineral enhancements might be suggested or endorsed by your PCP or dietitian, contingent upon the phase of your kidney ailment. Normally a well-adjusted eating routine will supply you with enough nutrients and minerals to keep you healthy. Be that as it may, dialysis treatment will wash some water-solvent nutrients out of your body.

At the point when you're on dialysis you should just take nutrient enhancements that have been suggested for you, as specific nutrients and minerals can be destructive. It's significant for you to counsel your primary care physician. Nutrients might be helpful to enhance your wellbeing when you have or experience any of the accompanying:

incessantly poor or flighty dietary patterns

diminished hunger, sickness, heaving

taste changes or nourishment abhorrences

unfortunate weight reduction

nourishment weakness

nutrient misfortune during dialysis.

KidneyVital means to enhance the key nutrients and follow components, to assist you with carrying on with a progressively dynamic life. It has been uniquely detailed by kidney masters to give the supplements your body needs and rejects those fixings that could be destructive to your wellbeing. Wholesome attributes of the five fundamental nutritional categories. Check this diagram beneath for the supplements and other critical segments in the fundamental nutritional categories.

What are kidney diseases and what causes them?

Kidney Diseases

By and large, kidney disappointment is brought about by other medical issues that have done lasting harm (hurt) to your kidneys gradually, after some time. At the point when your kidneys are harmed, they may not fill in just as they should. In the event·that the harm to your kidneys keeps on deteriorating and your kidneys are less and less ready to carry out their responsibility, you have incessant kidney sickness. Kidney disappointment is the last (most serious) phase of constant kidney malady. This is the reason kidney disappointment is likewise called end-organize renal sickness, or ESRD for short. Diabetes is the most well-known reason for ESRD. Hypertension is the second most normal reason for ESRD. Different issues that can cause kidney disappointment include:

Immune system ailments, for example, lupus and IgA nephropathy

Hereditary ailments (infections you are brought into the world with, for example, polycystic kidney ailment

Nephrotic disorder

Urinary tract issues

Here and there the kidneys can quit working abruptly (inside two days). This kind of kidney disappointment is called intense kidney damage or intense renal disappointment. Regular reasons for intense renal disappointment include:

Respiratory failure

Illicit medication uses and medication misuse

Insufficient blood streaming to the kidneys

Urinary tract issues

This kind of kidney disappointment isn't constantly changeless. Your kidneys may return to typical or practically ordinary with treatment and in the event that you don't have different genuine medical issues. Having one of the medical issues that can prompt kidney disappointment doesn't imply that you will have kidney disappointment. Carrying on with a solid way of life and working with your PCP to control these medical issues can enable your kidneys to work for whatever length of time that conceivable.

Symptoms of Kidney diseases

Incessant kidney infection (CKD) normally deteriorates gradually, and side effects may not show up until your kidneys are gravely harmed. In the late phases of CKD, as you are nearing kidney disappointment (ESRD), you may see side effects that are brought about by waste and additional liquid structure up in your body.

You may see at least one of the accompanying manifestations if your kidneys are starting to come up short:

Tingling

Muscle issues

Queasiness and heaving

Not feeling hungry

Growing in your feet and lower legs

An excess of (pee) or insufficient pee

Issue resting

Issue resting

On the off chance that your kidneys quit working all of a sudden (intense kidney disappointment), you may see at least one of the accompanying indications:

Stomach (tummy) torment

Back torment

The runs

Fever

Nosebleeds

Rash

Retching

Having at least one of any of the manifestations above might be an indication of genuine kidney issues. On the off chance that you see any of these manifestations, you should contact your primary care physician immediately.

Treatment of Kidney Failure

On the off chance that you have kidney disappointment (end-organize renal ailment or ESRD), you will require dialysis or a kidney transplant to live. There is no remedy for ESRD, however numerous individuals live long lives while on dialysis or subsequent to having a kidney transplant.

Adjusting to Kidney Failure

Discovering that you have kidney disappointment can come as a stun, regardless of whether you have known for quite a while that your kidneys were not functioning admirably. Changing your way of life to set aside a few minutes for your medicines can make adapting to this new reality considerably harder. You may need to quit working or find better approaches to work out. You may feel dismal or apprehensive. All isn't lost. You can find support to feel good and have a satisfying life.

What are kidney diseases

The kidneys are a couple of clench hand measured organs situated at the base of the rib confine. There is one kidney on each side of the spine. Kidneys are fundamental to having a sound body. They are for the most part answerable for sifting waste items, overabundance water, and different debasements out of the blood. These poisons are put away in the bladder and afterward expelled during pee. The kidneys additionally direct pH, salt, and potassium levels in the body. They produce hormones that manage circulatory strain and control the creation of red platelets. The kidneys even initiate a type of nutrient D that enables the body to assimilate calcium.

Kidney malady influences roughly 26 million American grown-ups. It happens when your kidneys become harmed and can't play out their capacity. Harm might be brought about by diabetes, hypertension, and different other constant (long haul) conditions. Kidney malady can prompt other medical issues, including powerless bones, nerve harm, and lack of healthy sustenance.

On the off chance that the sickness deteriorates after some time, your kidneys may quit working totally. This implies dialysis will be required to play out the capacity of the kidneys. Dialysis is a treatment that channels and filters the blood utilizing a machine. It can't fix kidney ailment; however, it can drag out your life.

What are the sorts and reasons for kidney sickness?

Constant kidney illness

The most well-known type of kidney illness is incessant kidney infection. Incessant kidney sickness is a long-haul condition that doesn't improve after some time. It's ordinarily brought about by hypertension.

Hypertension is risky for the kidneys since it can press the glomeruli. Glomeruli are the small veins in the kidneys where blood is cleaned. After some time, the expanded weight harms these vessels and kidney capacity starts to decay.

Kidney capacity will in the end weaken to the point where the kidneys can never again play out their activity appropriately. For this situation, an individual would need to go on dialysis. Dialysis sift additional liquid and waste through of the blood. Dialysis can help treat kidney ailment yet it can't fix it. A kidney transplant might be another treatment choice relying upon your conditions.

Diabetes is likewise a significant reason for incessant kidney infection. Diabetes is a gathering of sicknesses that causes high glucose. The expanded degree of sugar in the blood harms the veins in the kidneys after some time. This implies the kidneys can't spotless the blood appropriately. Kidney disappointment can happen when your body winds up over-burden with poisons.

Kidney stones

Kidney stones are another regular kidney issue. They happen when minerals and different substances in the blood take shape in the kidneys, framing strong masses (stones). Kidney stones for the most part leave the body during pee. Passing kidney stones can be very difficult, however they once in a while cause critical issues.

Glomerulonephritis

Glomerulonephritis is an aggravation of the glomeruli. Glomeruli are very little structures inside the kidneys that channel the blood. Glomerulonephritis can be brought about by diseases, drugs, or inherent anomalies (issue that happen during or not long after birth). It frequently shows signs of improvement all alone.

Polycystic kidney ailment

Polycystic kidney ailment is a hereditary issue that causes various pimples (little sacs of liquid) to develop in the kidneys. These pimples can meddle with kidney capacity and cause kidney disappointment. (Note that individual kidney sores are genuinely normal and quite often innocuous. Polycystic kidney ailment is a different, progressively genuine condition.)

Urinary tract diseases

Urinary tract diseases (UTIs) are bacterial contaminations of any piece of the urinary framework. Diseases in the bladder and urethra are the most widely recognized. They are effectively treatable and seldom lead to more medical issues. Be that as it may, whenever left untreated, these diseases can spread to the kidneys and cause kidney disappointment.

What are the side effects of kidney ailment?

Kidney illness is a condition that can without much of a stretch go unnoticed until the manifestations become extreme. The accompanying manifestations are early cautioning signs that you may be creating kidney sickness:

exhaustion

trouble concentrating

issue dozing

poor hunger

muscle cramping

swollen feet/lower legs

puffiness around the eyes in the first part of the day

dry, layered skin

visit pee, particularly late around evening time

Find out additional: Kidney capacity tests »

Serious side effects that could mean your kidney illness is advancing into kidney disappointment include:

queasiness

retching

loss of craving

changes in pee yield

liquid maintenance

sickliness (a reduction in red platelets)

diminished sex drive

abrupt ascent in potassium levels (hyperkalemia)

irritation of the pericardium (liquid filled sac that covers the heart)

What are the hazard factors for creating kidney infection?

Individuals with diabetes have a higher danger of creating kidney infection. Diabetes is the main source of kidney ailment, representing around 44 percent of new cases. You may likewise be bound to get kidney infection in the event that you:

have hypertension

have other relatives with interminable kidney sickness are older are of African, Hispanic, Asian, or American Indian drop

How is kidney infection analyzed?

Your PCP will initially decide if you have a place in any of the high-hazard gatherings. They will at that point run a few tests to check whether your kidneys are working appropriately. These tests may include:

Glomerular filtration rate (GFR)

This test will quantify how well your kidneys are functioning and decide the phase of kidney illness.

Ultrasound or figured tomography (CT) Scan

Ultrasounds and CT sweeps produce clear pictures of your kidneys and urinary tract. The photos enable your PCP to check whether your kidneys are too little or enormous. They can likewise show any tumors or basic issues that might be available.

Kidney biopsy

During a kidney biopsy, your PCP will evacuate a little bit of tissue from your kidney while you're quieted. The tissue test can enable your primary care physician to decide the sort of kidney ailment you have and how a lot of harm has happened.

Pee test

Your primary care physician may demand a pee test to test for egg whites. Egg whites is a protein that can be passed into your pee when your kidneys are harmed.

Blood creatinine test

Creatinine is a waste item. It's discharged into the blood when creatine (a particle put away in muscle) is separated. The degrees of creatinine in your blood will increment if your kidneys aren't working appropriately.

Find out increasingly: Excessive pee around evening time »

How is kidney illness treated?

Treatment for kidney illness normally centers around controlling the basic reason for the ailment. This implies your PCP will assist you with bettering deal with your circulatory strain, glucose, and cholesterol levels. They may utilize at least one of the accompanying techniques to treat kidney malady.

Medications and medicine

Your PCP will either endorse angiotensin-changing over chemical (ACE) inhibitors, for example, lisinopril and ramipril, or angiotensin receptor blockers (ARBs, for example, irbesartan and olmesartan. These are pulse prescriptions that can slow the movement of kidney infection. Your primary care physician may recommend these drugs to safeguard kidney work, regardless of whether you don't have hypertension.

You may likewise be treated with cholesterol drugs, (for example, simvastatin). These prescriptions can diminish blood cholesterol levels and help keep up kidney wellbeing. Contingent upon your indications, your primary care physician may likewise recommend medications to diminish growing and treat paleness (decline in the quantity of red platelets).

Dietary and way of life changes

Making changes to your eating regimen is similarly as significant as taking drug. Embracing a sound way of life can help anticipate a large number of the basic reasons for kidney infection. Your primary care physician may suggest that you:

control diabetes through insulin infusions

cut back on nourishments high in cholesterol

cut back on salt

start a heart-sound eating regimen that incorporates crisp organic products, veggies, entire grains, and low-fat dairy items

limit liquor utilization

stop smoking

increment physical movement

get more fit

Dialysis and kidney ailment

Dialysis is a counterfeit technique for separating the blood. It's utilized when somebody's kidneys have fizzled or are near falling flat. Numerous individuals with late-arrange kidney ailment must go on dialysis for all time or until a giver kidney is found.

There are two sorts of dialysis: hemodialysis and peritoneal dialysis.

Hemodialysis

In hemodialysis, the blood is siphoned through a unique machine that channels out waste items and liquid. Hemodialysis is done at your home or in an emergency clinic or dialysis focus. The vast majority have three sessions for every week, with every session enduring three to five hours. Be that as it may, hemodialysis should likewise be possible in shorter, progressively visit sessions.

A little while before beginning hemodialysis, a great many people will have medical procedure to make an arteriovenous (AV) fistula. An AV fistula is made by associating a corridor and a vein just beneath the skin, regularly in the lower arm. The bigger vein enables an expanded measure of blood to stream consistently through the body during hemodialysis treatment. This implies more blood can be sifted and sanitized. An arteriovenous unite (a circled, plastic cylinder) might be embedded and utilized for a similar reason if a corridor and vein can't be combined.

The most well-known reactions of hemodialysis are low pulse, muscle cramping, and tingling.

Peritoneal dialysis

In peritoneal dialysis, the peritoneum (layer that lines the stomach divider) subs for the kidneys. A cylinder is embedded and used to fill the belly with a liquid called dialysate. Squander items in the blood stream from the peritoneum into the dialysate. The dialysate is then depleted from the midriff.

There are two types of peritoneal dialysis: persistent wandering peritoneal dialysis, where the stomach area is occupied and depleted a few times during the day, and nonstop cycler-helped peritoneal dialysis, which uses a machine to cycle the liquid all through the guts around evening time while the individual rests.

The most widely recognized reactions of peritoneal dialysis are contaminations in the stomach cavity or in the zone where the cylinder was embedded. Opposite symptoms may incorporate weight increase and hernias. A hernia is the point at which the digestive system pushes through a shaky area or tear in the lower stomach divider.

What is the long-haul standpoint for somebody with kidney sickness?

Kidney malady ordinarily doesn't leave once it's analyzed. The most ideal approach to keep up kidney wellbeing is to receive a solid way of life and pursue your primary care physician's recommendation. Kidney illness can deteriorate after some time. It might even prompt kidney disappointment. Kidney disappointment can be perilous whenever left untreated.

Kidney disappointment happens when your kidneys are scarcely working or not working by any stretch of the imagination. This is overseen by dialysis. Dialysis includes the utilization of a machine to channel squander from your blood. At times, your primary care physician may prescribe a kidney transplant.

In what manner can kidney malady be counteracted?

Some hazard factors for kidney sickness —, for example, age, race, or family ancestry — are difficult to control. In any case, there are measures you can take to help anticipate kidney infection:

drink a lot of water

control glucose in the event that you have diabetes

control circulatory strain

lessen salt admission

stop smoking

Be cautious with over-the-counter medications

You ought to consistently adhere to the measurement guidelines for over-the-counter prescriptions. Taking an excessive amount of headache medicine (Bayer) or ibuprofen (Advil, Motrin) can cause kidney harm. Call your primary care physician if the ordinary portions of these meds aren't controlling your agony successfully.

Get tried

Get some information about getting a blood test for kidney issues. Kidney issues for the most part don't cause side effects until they're further developed. A fundamental metabolic board (BMP) is a standard blood test that should be possible as a component of a normal therapeutic test. It checks your blood for creatinine or urea. These are synthetic compounds that break into the blood when the kidneys aren't working appropriately. A BMP can distinguish kidney issues early, when they're simpler to treat. You ought to be tried every year on the off chance that you have diabetes, coronary illness, or hypertension.

Farthest point certain nourishments

Various synthetic compounds in your nourishment can add to specific kinds of kidney stones. These include:

inordinate sodium

creature protein, for example, meat and chicken citrus extract, found in citrus natural products, for example, oranges, lemons, and grapefruits oxalate, a substance found in beets, spinach, sweet potatoes, and chocolate

Get some information about calcium

Converse with your PCP before taking a calcium supplement. Some calcium enhancements have been connected to an expanded danger of kidney stones.

More About Kidney Diseases

Kidney malady can influence your body's capacity to clean your blood, sift additional water through of your blood, and help control your circulatory strain. It can likewise influence red platelet creation and nutrient D digestion required for bone wellbeing. You're brought into the world with two kidneys. They're on either side of your spine, simply over your midriff.

At the point when your kidneys are harmed, squander items and liquid can develop in your body. That can cause expanding in your lower legs, queasiness, shortcoming, poor rest, and brevity of breath. Without treatment, the harm can deteriorate and your kidneys may in the long run quit working. That is not kidding, and it tends to be hazardous.

What Your Kidneys Do

Sound kidneys:

Keep a parity of water and minerals, (for example, sodium, potassium, and phosphorus) in your blood. Expel squander from your blood after processing, muscle movement, and introduction to synthetic compounds or drugs. Make renin, which your body uses to help deal with your circulatory strain. Make a synthetic called erythropoietin, which prompts your body to make red platelets. Make a functioning type of nutrient D, required for bone wellbeing and different things

Intense Kidney Problems

In the event that your kidneys all of a sudden quit working, specialists call it intense kidney damage or intense renal disappointment. The fundamental driver are:

Conditions That Affect Your Kidneys

Your kidneys help channel all the waste items your body develops in its characteristic procedures. Gain more from WebMD about the medicinal issues that can hurt them.

Insufficient blood stream to the kidneys

Direct harm to the kidneys themselves

Pee sponsored up in the kidneys

Those things can happen when you:

Have horrendous damage with blood misfortune, for example, in an auto wreck

Are dried out or your muscle tissue separates, sending an excess of protein into your circulatory system

Go into stun on the grounds that you have a serious contamination called sepsis

Have an expanded prostate that hinders your pee stream

Ingest certain medications or are around sure poisons that straightforwardly harm the kidney

Have inconveniences during a pregnancy, for example, eclampsia and pre-eclampsia

Immune system sicknesses, when your insusceptible framework assaults your body, can likewise cause intense kidney damage. Individuals with extreme heart or liver disappointment usually go into intense kidney damage, also.

Interminable Kidney Disease

At the point when your kidneys don't function admirably for longer than 3 months, specialists call it constant kidney sickness. You might not have any manifestations in the beginning times, yet that is the point at which it's more straightforward to treat.

Ten Signs you might be having kidney diseases

In excess of 37 million American grown-ups are living with kidney illness and most don't have any acquaintance with it. "There are various physical indications of kidney infection, yet some of the time individuals ascribe them to different conditions. Additionally, those with kidney ailment tend not to encounter side effects until the exceptionally late stages, when the kidneys are falling flat or when there are a lot of protein in the pee. This is one reason why just 10% of individuals with incessant kidney malady realize that they have it," says Dr. Joseph Vassalotti, Chief Medical Officer at the National Kidney Foundation. While the best way to know without a doubt in the event that you have kidney infection is to get tried, Dr. Vassalotti shares 10 potential signs you may have kidney infection. In case you're in danger for kidney illness because of hypertension, diabetes, a family ancestry of kidney disappointment or in case you're more seasoned than age 60, it's essential to get tried every year for kidney infection. Make certain to specify any manifestations you're encountering to your social insurance expert. You're progressively worn out, have less vitality or are experiencing difficulty concentrating. An extreme abatement in kidney capacity can prompt a development of poisons and pollutions in the blood. This can make individuals feel worn out, frail and can make it difficult to focus. Another confusion of kidney sickness is frailty, which can cause shortcoming and exhaustion. You're experiencing difficulty resting. At the point when the kidneys aren't sifting appropriately, poisons remain in the blood as opposed to leaving the body through the pee. This can make it hard to rest. There is likewise a connection among corpulence and interminable kidney illness, and rest apnea is progressively regular in those with incessant kidney infection, contrasted and the all-inclusive community.

You have dry and irritated skin. Sound kidneys do numerous significant occupations. They expel squanders and additional liquid from your body, help make red platelets, help keep bones solid and work to keep up the perfect measure of minerals in your blood. Dry and bothersome skin can be an indication of the mineral and bone sickness that frequently goes with cutting edge kidney malady, when the kidneys are never again ready to keep the correct equalization of minerals and supplements in your blood.

You want to pee all the more regularly. In the event that you want to pee all the more regularly, particularly around evening time, this can be an indication of kidney sickness. At the point when the kidneys channels are harmed, it can make an expansion in the inclination pee. Some of the time this can likewise be an indication of a urinary disease or amplified prostate in men. You see blood in your pee. Sound kidneys commonly keep the platelets in the body when sifting squanders from the blood to make pee, however when the kidney's channels have been harmed, these platelets can begin to "spill" out into the pee.

Notwithstanding flagging kidney malady, blood in the pee can be demonstrative of tumors, kidney stones or a disease.

Your pee is frothy. Inordinate air pockets in the pee – particularly those that expect you to flush a few times before they leave— demonstrate protein in the pee. This froth may resemble the froth you see when scrambling eggs, as the basic protein found in pee, egg whites, is a similar protein that is found in eggs.

You're encountering relentless puffiness around your eyes. Protein in the pee is an early sign that the kidneys' channels have been harmed, enabling protein to spill into the pee. This puffiness around your eyes can be because of the way that your kidneys are releasing a lot of protein in the pee, as opposed to keeping it in the body.

Your lower legs and feet are swollen. Diminished kidney capacity can prompt sodium maintenance, causing expanding in your feet and lower legs. Growing in the lower furthest points can likewise be an indication of coronary illness, liver sickness and constant leg vein issues.

You have a poor hunger. This is an exceptionally broad side effect, however a development of poisons coming about because of diminished kidney capacity can be one of the causes.

Your muscles are cramping. Electrolyte uneven characters can result from hindered kidney work. For instance, low calcium levels and inadequately controlled phosphorus may add to muscle cramping.

Why does the renal diet work?

Renal diet works because the shape of the body along with the digestion is totally effective in this regard for the body and following are the steps that are followed for the better work of the renal diet.

Eating Right for Chronic Kidney Disease

You may need to change what you eat to deal with your ceaseless kidney illness (CKD). Work with an enlisted dietitian to build up a supper plan that incorporates nourishments that you appreciate eating while at the same time keeping up your kidney wellbeing.

The means underneath will assist you with eating directly as you deal with your kidney ailment. The initial three stages (1-3) are significant for all individuals with kidney ailment. The last two stages (4-5) may wind up significant as your kidney capacity goes down.

The initial steps to eating right

Stage 1: Choose and plan nourishments with less salt and sodium

Why? To help control your circulatory strain. You're eating regimen ought to contain under 2,300 milligrams of sodium every day. Purchase new nourishment frequently. Sodium (a piece of salt) is added to many arranged or bundled nourishments you purchase at the general store or at eateries. Cook nourishments without any preparation as opposed to eating arranged nourishments, "quick" nourishments, solidified meals, and canned food sources that are higher in sodium. At the point when you set up your very own nourishment, you control what goes into it.

Use flavors, herbs, and sans sodium seasonings instead of salt.

Check for sodium on the Nutrition Facts mark of nourishment bundles. A Daily Value of 20 percent or more means the nourishment is high in sodium. Attempt lower-sodium renditions of solidified meals and other comfort nourishments. Wash canned vegetables, beans, meats, and fish with water before eating.

Stage 2: Eat the perfect sum and the correct sorts of protein

Why? To help ensure your kidneys. At the point when your body utilizes protein, it produces squander. Your kidneys evacuate this waste. Eating more protein than you need may make your kidneys work more enthusiastically. Eat little parts of protein nourishments.

Protein is found in nourishments from plants and creatures. The vast majority eat the two kinds of protein. Converse with your dietitian about how to pick the correct mix of protein nourishments for you.

Creature protein nourishments:

Chicken

Fish

Meat

Eggs

Dairy

A cooked bit of chicken, fish, or meat is around 2 to 3 ounces or about the size of a deck of cards. A bit of dairy nourishments is ½ cup of milk or yogurt, or one cut of cheddar.

Plant-protein nourishments:

Beans

Nuts

Grains

A segment of cooked beans is about ½ cup, and a segment of nuts is ¼ cup. A bit of bread is solitary cut, and a part of cooked rice or cooked noodles is ½ cup.

Stage 3: Choose nourishments that are solid for your heart

Why? To assist keep with fatting from working up in your veins, heart, and kidneys. To assist keep with fatting from working up in your veins, heart, and kidneys.

Flame broil, sear, heat, dish, or pan-fried food nourishments, rather than profound fricasseeing.

Cook with nonstick cooking shower or a limited quantity of olive oil rather than spread.

Cut back excess from meat and expel skin from poultry before eating.

Attempt to constrain soaked and trans fats. Peruse the nourishment name.

Heart-solid nourishments:

Lean cuts of meat, for example, midsection or round

Poultry without the skin

Fish

Beans

Vegetables

Organic products

Low-fat or sans fat milk, yogurt, and cheddar

Farthest point liquor

Drink liquor just with some restraint: close to one beverage for each day on the off chance that you are a lady, and close to two in the event that you are a man. Drinking a lot of liquor can harm the liver, heart, and cerebrum and cause genuine medical issues. Ask your social insurance supplier how much liquor you can drink securely.

The subsequent stages to eating right

As your kidney capacity goes down, you may need to eat nourishments with less phosphorus and potassium. Your social insurance supplier will utilize lab tests to check phosphorus and potassium levels in your blood, and you can work with your dietitian to change your feast plan. More data is given in the NIDDK wellbeing point, Nutrition for Advanced Chronic Kidney Disease.

Stage 4: Choose nourishments and beverages with less phosphorus

Why? To help ensure your bones and veins. At the point when you have CKD, phosphorus can develop in your blood. A lot of phosphorus in your blood pulls calcium from your bones, making your bones slender, frail, and bound to break. Significant levels of phosphorus in your blood can likewise cause irritated skin, and bone and joint agony.

Many bundled nourishments have included phosphorus. Search for phosphorus—or for words with "PHOS"— on fixing names.

Shop meats and some new meat and poultry can have included phosphorus. Request that the butcher assist you with picking crisp meats without included phosphorus.

Nourishments Lower in Phosphorus

Crisp products of the soil

Breads, pasta, rice

Rice milk (not advanced)

Corn and rice oats

Light-hued soft drinks/pop, for example, lemon-lime or natively constructed frosted tea

Nourishments Higher in Phosphorus

Meat, poultry, fish

Wheat grains and cereal

Dairy nourishments

Beans, lentils, nuts

Dim shaded soft drinks/pop, fruit juice, some packaged or canned frosted teas that have included phosphorus

Your social insurance supplier may converse with you about taking a phosphate folio with dinners to bring down the measure of phosphorus in your blood. A phosphate fastener is a drug that demonstrations like a wipe to absorb, or tie, phosphorus while it is in the stomach. Since it is bound, the phosphorus doesn't get into your blood. Rather, your body expels the phosphorus through your stool.

Stage 5: Choose nourishments with the perfect measure of potassium

Why? To support your nerves and muscles work the correct way. Issues can happen when blood potassium levels are excessively high or excessively low. Harmed kidneys enable potassium to develop in your blood, which can cause genuine heart issues. Your nourishment and drink decisions can assist you with bringing down your potassium level, if necessary.

Salt substitutes can be exceptionally high in potassium. Peruse the fixing mark. Check with your supplier about utilizing salt substitutes.

Channel canned products of the soil before eating.

Nourishments Lower in Potassium

Apples, peaches

Carrots, green beans

White bread and pasta

White rice

Rice milk (not improved)

Cooked rice and wheat grains, corn meal

Apple, grape, or cranberry juice

Nourishments Higher in Potassium

Oranges, bananas, and squeezed orange

Potatoes, tomatoes

Dark colored and wild rice

Grain oats

Dairy nourishments

Entire wheat bread and pasta

Beans and nuts

A few drugs additionally can raise your potassium level. Your social insurance supplier may alter the meds you take.

What are renal diet benefits?

There are many benefits of renal diet as it bolsters vitamin C supplementation.

The significance of satisfactory nutrient C, or ascorbic corrosive, as a cell reinforcement and in collagen amalgamation is settled; be that as it may, there are extraordinary worries with respect to keeping away from over the top sums in CKD. Current proposals for support hemodialysis (MHD) patients exhort supplementation with ascorbic corrosive 75-90 mg every day (Nephrol Dial Transplant. 2007;22[Suppl 2]:ii45-ii87) to supplant the misfortunes of this water-dissolvable nutrient that happen during dialysis. This measure of nutrient C is found in most renal multivitamins, i.e., nutrient blends endorsed explicitly to require the necessities of MHD patients, however evaluates from the Dialysis Outcomes and Practice Patterns Study (DOPPS) demonstrate that renal multivitamins are recommended for just about

70% of dialysis patients in the United States (Am J Kidney Dis. 2004; 44[5 Suppl 2]:61-67).

With respect to advantages of renal multivitamin use, the creators report that "patients taking such nutrients had a 16% lower mortality hazard than patients not taking water-dissolvable nutrients, after modification for age, sex, race, comorbid conditions, hemoglobin, serum egg whites, weight record, time on HD, normal office single-pool Kt/V, and normal office standardized protein catabolic rate." Since dietary wellsprings of nutrient C are frequently limited in view of worries about potassium, an everyday renal multivitamin can be a significant piece of standard consideration for dialysis patients. Since nutrient C is discharged by the kidney, consumption more noteworthy than 100-200 mg/day ought to be stayed away from in CKD to maintain a strategic distance from oxalosis, which is the gathering of the metabolic result of ascorbic corrosive. Numerous organs and tissues of the body can be influenced by oxalate stores, including the kidneys. Instances of intense renal disappointment (ARF) have been reported. As of late, Nankivell and Murali detailed oxalosis bringing about unite disappointment in a kidney transplant beneficiary who had been taking self-endorsed dosages of nutrient C 2,000 mg every day as a dialysis tolerant for the three years before transplant (N Engl J Med. 2008;358:e4).

So also, a case report by McHugh and partners (Anaesth Intensive Care. 2008;36:585-588) portrays mortality from nutrient C-actuated ARF. Oxalosis was affirmed on post-mortem in this patient, who, unbeknownst to doctors, had been ingesting "a few grams for every day" of nutrient C in the conviction that it would be useful for his wellbeing.

Movement to renal parenchymal harm and end-organize renal illness, which is by all accounts to a great extent free of the underlying affront, is the last basic pathway for ceaseless, proteinuric nephropathies in creatures and people. The key occasion is upgraded glomerular hairlike weight; this weakens glomerular penetrability to proteins and licenses unreasonable measures of proteins to arrive at the lumen of the proximal tubule. The optional procedure of reabsorption of sifted proteins can add to renal interstitial damage by enacting intracellular occasions, including upregulation of the qualities encoding vasoactive and fiery go betweens. Both interstitial irritation and movement of malady can be constrained by such medications as angiotensin-changing over catalyst inhibitors, which reinforce the glomerular porousness obstruction to proteins and in this manner limit proteinuria and separated protein-subordinate provocative sign. Clinical information firmly propose that abatement would now be able to be accomplished in certain patients with constant renal infection. On account of the momentum slack time between beginning treatment and reduction, be that as it may, a significant extent of patients still progresses to end-arrange renal sickness before renal capacity starts to settle. A multimodal approach that focuses on lessening or evacuating all hazard components related with the movement of renal infection may diminish the opportunity to reduction of the ailment for most patients with proteinuric nephropathies.

Cardiovascular and renal advantages of dry bean and soybean consumption

Dry beans and soybeans are supplement thick, fiber-rich, and are top notch wellsprings of protein. Defensive and restorative impacts of both dry bean and soybean admission have been reported. Studies show that dry bean admission can possibly diminish serum cholesterol focuses, improve numerous parts of the diabetic state, and give metabolic advantages that guide in weight control. Soybeans are a novel wellspring of the isoflavones genistein and diadzein, which have various organic capacities. Soybeans and soyfoods conceivably have multifaceted wellbeing advancing impacts, including cholesterol decrease, improved vascular wellbeing, saved bone mineral thickness, and decrease of menopausal side effects. Soy seems to effectsly affect renal capacity, in spite of the fact that these impacts are not surely known. Though populaces devouring high admissions of soy have lower prevalences of specific malignancies, conclusive test information are deficient to explain a defensive job of soy. The accessibility of vegetable items and assets is expanding, fusing dry beans and soyfoods into the eating routine can be down to earth and pleasant. With the move toward a more plant-based eating routine, dry beans and soy will be powerful instruments in the treatment and aversion of incessant illness.

Benefits of Renal Diet

To build up if the advantage of angiotensin changing over compound inhibitor treatment in hindering dynamic diabetic renal damage is because of a particular intrarenal impact of the fundamental hypotensive impact, we examined the impact of long haul ramipril treatment on circulatory strain, glomerular filtration rate, and urinary protein discharge in streptozotocin-diabetic precipitously hypertensive rodents. The hypotensive impact of ramipril was counteracted by a high salt eating regimen, which didn't adjust the level of renal angiotensin changing over compound hindrance. Three weeks after uninephrectomy and enlistment of diabetes, rodents were apportioned to three gatherings. Gatherings 1 and 2 were given 1% NaCl, though bunch 3 was given water as drinking arrangement. Multi week later, bunches 2 and 3 got 0.4 mg/kg/day ramipril in their drinking arrangement, which was proceeded over a 2-month time span. Ramipril delivered a circulatory strain fall just in water-drinking rodents (bunch 3) in spite of a comparable decrease in plasma and renal angiotensin changing over compound movement in bunches 2 and 3. Salt-stacked rodents had a dynamic increment in urinary protein discharge over the span of study. Ramipril treatment forestalled an expansion in protein discharge just in creatures given water and with a decreased systolic pulse. Glomerular filtration rate was comparable in every one of the three gatherings. Ramipril treatment improved creature endurance autonomously of a decrease in circulatory strain or an impact on proteinuria. In spite of the fact that it is conceivable that angiotensin changing over catalyst inhibitors have explicit intrarenal impacts lessening movement of diabetic proteinuria, accompanying control of foundational circulatory strain has all the earmarks of being important to exhibit an advantage.

The renal benefits of a healthy life style

The renal advantages of a solid way of life Over the following decade, the quantity of patients with end-organize renal sickness requiring treatment by dialysis may twofold, and even created countries will experience issues adapting to this disturbing increment. There is a pressing need to feature the significance of modifiable hazard factors as a reason for treatment procedures to counteract the advancement and movement of constant kidney infection (CKD). This should incorporate dynamic augmentation of our present comprehension of a sound way of life.

Stoutness has turned into a universal plague, and adjusting this pestilence by changing way of life components is urgent to wellbeing and to the anticipation of kidney ailment today and later on. Liquor may effectsly affect renal capacity like those related with cardiovascular malady; nonetheless, liquor utilization is likewise a potential hazard factor for the advancement of glomerular harm, hypertension, and hypertensive nephrosclerosis. In patients with diabetes, smoking expands the danger of creating nephropathy and advancing to end-organize renal disappointment. Smoking likewise decreases renal capacity and builds albuminuria or proteinuria in the all-inclusive community. Dietary salt admission influences renal capacity through its consequences for pulse and fibrosis, perhaps by means of tumor development factor-β1–subordinate pathways, proposing that unnecessary salt admission might be a significant direct pathogenic factor for cardiovascular and renal ailment. Exercise decreases resting circulatory strain and avoids strange increments in pulse during physical effort. Humble weight reduction through diet and physical movement diminishes the frequency of type 2 diabetes in high-hazard people. The monetary weight forced by the expenses of dialysis and the high mortality identified with CKD presents a convincing contention for actualizing a savvy preventive methodology against end-arrange renal infection. To counteract CKD, proposals about a sound way of life went for the individual ought to be predictable with general wellbeing suggestions.

Interminable KIDNEY DISEASE AS AN EPIDEMIC PROBLEM

The overall increment in the quantity of patients with interminable kidney sickness (CKD) and subsequent end-organize renal ailment (ESRD) requiring renal substitution treatment is taking steps to arrive at pestilence extents throughout the following decade. ESRD profoundly affects grimness, mortality, and personal satisfaction, and forces a considerable weight on social insurance expenditure1. The scourge increment in the frequency of ESRD in numerous nations features the significance of the modifiable hazard factors as a reason for contriving treatment procedures to counteract the advancement and movement of CKD.

Endeavors to control the scourge of CKD and its cardiovascular difficulties have customarily centered around pharmacologic treatment of diabetes, hypertension, the lipid profile, and proteinuria2. CKD counteractive action and control systems incorporate characterizing in danger populaces and clarifying potential focuses for intercession. This should incorporate dynamic augmentation of our present comprehension of medicinal services and financial hazard factors.

Weight

Weight has turned into a universal plague, and there is developing understanding that specific way of life components is driving this pandemic. The cutting-edge way of life will in general support overconsumption and demoralizes consumption of vitality. Minor holes to be decided of vitality utilization and consumption lead to progressive yet enduring weight gain, and readdressing these patterns is essential to wellbeing and to counteracting kidney ailment today and in the future3.

The metabolic disorder, which is described by heftiness, insulin opposition, hyperinsulinemia, and dyslipidemia, might add to renal illness by numerous pathways, including the advancement of type 2 diabetes, hypertension, and cardiovascular malady. Corpulent patients can create proteinuria, which is trailed by dynamic loss of renal capacity in a generous extent of cases. Weight related glomerulopathy (ORG) is unmistakable from idiopathic central and segmental glomerulosclerosis (FSGS), and has a lower occurrence of nephrotic disorder, increasingly sluggish course, reliable nearness of glomerulomegaly, and milder foot process combination. The 10-overlay increment of ORG in rate in the course of recent years recommends a recently developing epidemic4.

Renal biopsies and post-mortem studies have indicated that FSGS causes the most well-known types of histologic injuries in corpulent patients with proteinuria. Extensive information show that hyperinsulinemia can intervene glomerular injury5, albeit glomerular hyperfiltration, hyperlipidemia, leptin, and resistin, a hormone discharged by adipocytes, may likewise be engaged with the pathogenesis of FSGS related with obesity6.

Weight reduction diminishes proteinuria in patients with ORG. Praga et al contemplated a gathering of patients with heftiness related proteinuria that was treated with hypocaloric abstains from food more than 1 year, and announced a mean weight reduction of 12% and a diminishing in proteinuria >80%7. In another investigation of 30 overweight patients, a mean weight reduction of 4% was trailed by a 31% diminishing in proteinuria8.

When all is said in done, being overweight is related with a 2-to 6-overlap increment in the danger of hypertension. Clinical preliminaries have additionally indicated that weight reduction is compelling in the essential avoidance of hypertension and in the decrease of both systolic and diastolic circulatory strain in patients with typical or high blood pressure9. Diminishing the pervasiveness of corpulence by improving way of life components should help in the essential counteractive action of CKD, especially in created nations. We tentatively concentrated a gathering of 35 beefy beyond belief patients (29 ladies and 6 men; mean weight file 47.6 ± 5.9 kg/m2) with stoutness related proteinuria who had been treated by biliopancreatic redirection.

Liquor

At present, epidemiologic examinations have revealed that moderate liquor and wine admission have defensive effects10. Liquor may helpfully influence renal capacity through comparable components to those revealed for cardiovascular illness, for example, by adjusting blood high-thickness lipoproteins, fibrinogen, insulin, and hemostatic elements. Burchfiel et al11 found that liquor admission was contrarily connected with a raised level of renal arteriolar hyalinization, autonomous of other cardiovascular hazard factors at post-mortem.

In any case, liquor may have both positive and negative consequences for renal capacity. Liquor utilization is a potential hazard factor for glomerular harm, hypertension, and hypertensive nephrosclerosis12. In exploratory examinations, liquor bolstered creatures have altogether lower renal capacity and more interstitial edema than their isocaloric controls13. A case-control concentrate dependent on self-reports found that normal utilization of in excess of 2 mixed beverages for each day was related with an expanded danger of kidney disappointment in the general population14. Interestingly, a forthcoming investigation of 1658 medical caretakers tried out the Nurses' Health Study found no relationship between moderate liquor utilization and pace of decrease in renal function15.

SMOKING AS A RENAL RISK FACTOR

Diabetologists were the first to perceive the unfavorable impacts of smoking on the kidney. In individuals with either type 1 or type 2 diabetes, smoking expands the danger of creating nephropathy and about pairs the pace of movement to end-arrange renal failure16. Smoking builds circulatory strain, tachycardia, convergences of catecholamines, and renovascular obstruction, which is joined by diminishes in glomerular filtration rate (GFR) and filtration portion. The impacts of smoking are ventured to be brought about by nicotine itself in light of the fact that these unfriendly impacts are not related with smoking sans nicotine cigarettes17. In subjects without renal infection, backhanded proof focuses to particular afferent vasoconstriction, which ought to ensure the glomerular microcirculation against the ascent in fundamental circulatory strain. Conversely, in patients with essential renal ailment, the intense increment in pulse isn't reliably joined by afferent vasoconstriction. It has been contended that in interminable smokers, compensatory initiation of nitric oxide–subordinate vasodilation neutralizes smoking-prompted vasoconstriction.

To research in the case of smoking is identified with albuminuria and unusual renal capacity in nondiabetic people, Pinto-Sietsma et al18 contemplated 7476 members in the Prevention of Renal and Vascular End Stage Disease Study. Current smokers (≤20 or >20 cigarettes/day) and previous smokers had expanded middle egg whites discharge, and were bound to have high-ordinary albuminuria and microalbuminuria than nonsmokers. The level of members with a raised GFR was lower in previous smokers than in current smokers, and more prominent than in nonsmokers. Interestingly, the level of members with a diminished GFR was comparative in previous smokers and nonsmokers and fundamentally lower in previous smokers than in current smokers.

In a review case-control investigation of 4142 nondiabetic members 65 years old or more established in the Cardiovascular Health Study Cohort study, Bleyer et al19 found that the quantity of cigarettes smoked every day anticipated the decrease in renal capacity. This information propose that stopping smoking could diminish the danger of renal inadequacy in this more seasoned age gathering, which concurs with information from an investigation of 455 grown-ups in Minnesota that demonstrated that the reduction in creatinine freedom was more prominent in ex-smokers and ebb and flow smokers than in nonsmokers20. These examinations recommend that smoking decreases renal capacity and builds albuminuria or proteinuria in the all-inclusive community, a significant issue from a general wellbeing point of view.

Smoking is an incredible indicator of microalbuminuria in patients with essential hypertension. The commonness of microalbuminuria in lean, hypertensive smokers is almost twofold that in nonsmokers21. In an imminent investigation of variables anticipating the loss of renal capacity, Regalado et al22 distinguished smoking as the most dominant indicator in patients with essential hypertension however no proof of essential renal malady. Smoking may clarify at any rate some portion of the perception that patients with essential hypertension show a dynamic decay of renal capacity in spite of satisfactory control of blood pressure23.

Cigarette smoking speaks to a significant factor related with the movement of nephropathy in patients treated for hypertension and type 1 diabetes16. Absolutely, there are numerous valid justifications to quit smoking, especially for diabetic patients. Sawicki et al24 found that patients with type 1 diabetes and nephropathy who had great glycemic and circulatory strain control and had quit smoking had altogether lower danger of movement than current smokers. Male patients with glomerulonephritis25 or atherosclerotic ischemic nephropathy and who smoke26 are at expanded danger of hindered renal capacity.

Kasiske et al27 inspected the commonness and clinical connects of cigarette smoking in a huge accomplice of renal transplant beneficiaries. Contrasted and smoking under 25 pack-years or having never smoked, smoking in excess of 25 pack-years at transplantation was related with a 30% higher danger of join disappointment and an expanded danger of death. The impacts of smoking seem to disperse 5 years in the wake of stopping, recommending that more noteworthy exertion to urge patients to stop smoking before transplantation may diminish bleakness and mortality.

SALT INTAKE

The impact of salt on renal capacity is identified with both hypertension and to an immediate impact on renal capacity. Hypertension is both a reason and result of renal disappointment, yet the exact nature and commonness of hypertensive nephrosclerosis as a reason for renal disappointment stays disputable. There is solid proof that hypertension quickens the movement of exploratory renal infection and that control of pulse anticipates this movement. The connection between circulatory strain and ensuing renal infection gives off an impression of being certain and nonstop all through the full scope of pulse. In a 20-year network based, imminent, observational investigation of the relationship between hypertension on the future danger of CKD in 23,534 people, Haroun et al found a solid reviewed connection between CKD hazard and the Sixth Report of the Joint National Committee on Detection, Evaluation and Treatment of High Blood Pressure criteria for circulatory strain that was similarly solid in ladies as in men28.

Albeit epidemiologic information shows an immediate connection between dietary sodium admission and circulatory strain at the populace level, a few specialists question the all-inclusiveness of the discoveries and restrict general wellbeing proposals to diminish sodium consumption in the overall public. Results from creature ponders, epidemiologic examinations, and clinical preliminaries have demonstrated that a high admission of salt unfavorably influences circulatory strain. The DASH-Sodium preliminary tried the impacts on circulatory strain of 3 degrees of sodium: higher (focus of roughly 143 mmol/day, reflecting run of the mill U.S. utilization), middle of the road (focus of 106 mmol/day, mirroring the maximum furthest reaches of current U.S. suggestions), and lower (focus of 65 mmol/day). The information indicated that diminishing sodium admission diminished pulse in members with or without hypertension, which supports the present proposals to lower salt intake29,30.

A high salt admission might be applicable to the pathogenesis of fundamental hypertension and, free of its hypertensinogenic impacts, may create reactions in the kidney that lead to renal fibrosis, conceivably through expanded renal generation of tumor development factor (TGF)- β. Yu et al31 detailed the impact of a typical (1%) or high (8%) sodium chloride diet on myocardial and renal fibrosis in unexpectedly hypertensive rodents and normotensive Wistar-Kyoto rodents. High dietary salt prompted far reaching fibrosis and expanded TGF-β1 in the heart and kidney of normotensive and hypertensive rodents. These outcomes propose that dietary salt specifically affects fibrosis, conceivably by means of TGF-β1—subordinate pathways, and further recommend that over the top salt admission might be a significant direct pathogenic factor for cardiovascular and renal infection. Such information fortifies the present rules to constrain salt admission to 6 g/day.

PHYSICAL ACTIVITY

Inactive conduct is one of the most grounded hazard factors for some ceaseless illnesses and conditions, including cardiovascular sickness, hypertension, diabetes, heftiness, osteoporosis, colon malignant growth, renal infection, and sorrow. An ongoing audit of observational examinations announced that the hazard for all-cause mortality was 20% to 30% lower among grown-ups who met the Healthy People 2010 suggestions (30 minutes of moderate movement for at least 5 days of the week or 20 minutes of energetic action at least

3 times each week), and fairly lower for grown-ups who practiced tolerably or vivaciously at any rate a couple of times each month or once per week32.

Physical inertia is a significant hazard factor for cardiovascular ailment, and people who are less dynamic or physically fit have a 30% to half more serious hazard for hypertension. Together with diabetes mellitus, blood vessel hypertension is the most significant reason for renal disappointment and dialysis in created nations. The wellbeing and viability of gentle to direct exercise have noteworthy positive clinical ramifications for every single hypertensive patient. The activity actuated decrease in resting circulatory strain and counteractive action of irregular increments in pulse during physical effort lessens the danger of cardiovascular occasions. These progressions may likewise diminish the requirement for, and the expense and reactions of, antihypertensive medicine, and may improve personal satisfaction.

Easing back the movement of constant renal disappointment: Economic advantages and patients' points of view

In view of the anticipated increment in end-arrange renal malady (ESRD) rate (anticipated increment from 1998 to 2010; 86,825 to 172,667), pervasiveness (anticipated increment from 1998 to 2010; 326,217 to 661,330), and cost (complete cost dependent on 1998 proportion of Medicare versus non-Medicare cost; $16.74 billion of every 1998 to $39.35 billion out of 2010), a firm national exertion is expected to create procedures to slow the movement of constant renal disappointment (CRF). The inquiry emerges to how a lot of decrease in the movement of CRF would prompt an important reduction in the commonness and cost of ESRD. There are no target information that show the financial effect of easing back the movement of CRF. We built up a scientific model to evaluate the monetary effect of diminishing the movement of CRF by 10%, 20%, and 30%. US Renal Data System (USRDS) projections were utilized to demonstrate the pace of increment in ESRD frequency and pervasiveness. Glomerular filtration rate (GFR) at the commencement of ESRD treatment and cost per persistent year depended on USRDS information. The normal decrease in GFR in subjects with CRF was assessed to be 7.56 mL/min/y. All dollar reserve funds reflect 1998 expenses, limited for the future at 3% per annum. We likewise decided how a lot of easing back of the movement of CRF is significant from patients' points of view by methods for a composed survey (which asked about ability to go on a limited eating regimen, take six additional drugs for every day, and make six additional office visits for every year) and count of the pre-ESRD time picked up for various degrees of decrease in the movement of CRF. On the off chance that the pace of decrease in GFR diminished by 10%, 20%, and 30% after December 31, 1999, in all patients with GFRs of 60 mL/min or less, total direct human services investment funds through 2010 would approach roughly $18.56, $39.02, and $60.61 billion, individually. For a 10%, 20%, and 30% diminishing in the pace of decrease in GFR in all patients with a GFR of 30 mL/min or less, assessed total reserve funds through 2010 equivalent $9.06, $19.98, and $33.37 billion, separately. Reactions to the poll indicated that around 79% of subjects with CRF (n = 113) saw half a month's sans dialysis period noteworthy (P ≤ 0.0001), a period relating to a 10% decrease in the pace of decrease in GFR. Our information propose that the combined monetary effect of easing back the movement of CRF, even by as meager as 10%, would stun. They give solid help to the improvement and usage of concentrated reno-defensive endeavors starting at the beginning periods of constant renal illness and proceeded all through its course.

What you can eat and what is forbidden in the renal diet

Foods that are forbidden in the renal diet are as follows:

Dull Colored Colas

Notwithstanding the calories and sugar that colas give, they likewise contain added substances that contain phosphorus, particularly dull hued colas. Numerous nourishment producers include phosphorus during the preparing of nourishment and drinks to upgrade enhance, draw out timeframe of realistic usability and counteract staining. This additional phosphorus is significantly more absorbable by the human body than regular, creature or plant-based phosphorus (5Trusted Source). In contrast to common phosphorus, phosphorus as added substances isn't bound to protein. Or maybe, it's found as salt and exceptionally absorbable by the intestinal tract (6Trusted Source).

Added substance phosphorus can normally be found in an item's fixing rundown. Be that as it may, nourishment producers are not required to list the careful measure of added substance phosphorus on the nourishment mark. While added substance phosphorus substance changes relying upon the sort of cola, most dull hued colas are accepted to contain 50–100 mg in a 200-ml serving (7Trusted Source). Therefore, colas, particularly those dim in shading, ought to be evaded on a renal eating routine.

Avocados

Avocados are frequently touted for their numerous nutritious characteristics, including their heart-sound fats, fiber and cell reinforcements. While avocados are normally a sound expansion to the eating regimen, people with kidney infection may need to stay away from them. This is on the grounds that avocados are an exceptionally rich wellspring of potassium. One cup (150 grams) of avocado gives an astounding 727 mg of potassium (8). That is twofold the measure of potassium than a medium banana gives. In this way, avocados, including guacamole, ought to be kept away from on a renal eating routine, particularly on the off chance that you have been advised to watch your potassium admission.

Canned Foods

Canned nourishments, for example, soups, vegetables and beans, are regularly acquired as a result of their ease and comfort. Be that as it may, most canned nourishments contain high measures of sodium, as salt is added as an additive to build its timeframe of realistic usability (9Trusted Source). In view of the measure of sodium found in canned products, it's frequently prescribed that individuals with kidney ailment maintain a strategic distance from or limit their utilization.

Picking lower-sodium assortments or those named "no salt included" is ordinarily best. Also, depleting and flushing canned nourishments, for example, canned beans and fish, can diminish the sodium content by 33–80%, contingent upon the item

Entire Wheat Bread

Picking the correct bread can be mistaking for people with kidney ailment. Frequently for sound people, entire wheat bread is normally suggested over refined, white flour bread. Entire wheat bread might be a progressively nutritious decision, for the most part because of its higher fiber content. Be that as it may, white bread is typically suggested over entire wheat assortments for people with kidney sickness. This is a direct result of its phosphorus and potassium content. The more wheat and entire grains in the bread, the higher the phosphorus and potassium substance. For instance, a 1-ounce (30-gram) serving of entire wheat bread contains around 57 mg of phosphorus and 69 mg of potassium. In examination, white bread contains just 28 mg of both phosphorus and potassium (11, 12). Note that most bread and bread items, paying little heed to being white or entire wheat, additionally contain generally high measures of sodium (13Trusted Source). It's ideal to look at nourishment names of different sorts of bread, pick a lower-sodium choice, if conceivable, and screen your part estimates.

Dark colored Rice

Like entire wheat bread, dark colored rice is an entire grain that has a higher potassium and phosphorus content than its white rice partner. One cup of cooked darker rice contains 150 mg of phosphorus and 154 mg of potassium, while one cup of cooked white rice contains just 69 mg of phosphorus and 54 mg of potassium (14, 15). You might have the option to fit dark colored rice into a renal eating routine, yet just if the segment is controlled and offset with different nourishments to maintain a strategic distance from exorbitant every day admission of potassium and phosphorus. Bulgur, buckwheat, pearled grain and couscous are nutritious, lower-phosphorus grains that can make a decent substitute for dark colored rice.

Bananas

Bananas are known for their high potassium content. While they're normally low in sodium, one medium banana gives 422 mg of potassium (16). It might be hard to keep your every day potassium admission to 2,000 mg if a banana is a day by day staple. Shockingly, numerous other tropical organic products have high potassium substance also. Be that as it may, pineapples contain considerably less potassium than other tropical products of the soil be an increasingly appropriate, yet scrumptious, elective (17).

Dairy

Dairy items are plentiful in different nutrients and supplements. They're additionally a characteristic wellspring of phosphorus and potassium and a decent wellspring of protein. For instance, 1 cup (8 liquid ounces) of entire milk gives 222 mg of phosphorus and 349 mg of potassium (18). However, devouring an excessive amount of dairy, related to different phosphorus-rich nourishments, can be unfavorable to bone wellbeing in those with kidney sickness. This may sound astonishing, as milk and dairy are regularly prescribed for solid bones and muscle wellbeing. Be that as it may, when the kidneys are harmed, an excessive amount of phosphorus utilization can cause a development of phosphorus in the blood. This can make your bones slight and powerless after some time and increment the danger of bone breakage or crack (19Trusted Source). Dairy items are additionally high in protein. One cup (8 liquid ounces) of entire milk gives around 8 grams of protein (18).

Oranges and Orange Juice

While oranges and squeezed orange are seemingly most notable for their nutrient C substance, they are likewise rich wellsprings of potassium. One enormous orange (184 grams) gives 333 mg of potassium. Also, there are 473 mg of potassium in one cup (8 liquid ounces) of squeezed orange (20, 21). Given their potassium substance, oranges and squeezed orange likely should be maintained a strategic distance from or restricted on a renal eating routine. Grapes, apples and cranberries, just as their individual juices, are largely great substitutes for oranges and squeezed orange, as they have lower potassium substance.It might be critical to constrain dairy admission to dodge the development of protein squander in the blood. Dairy options like unenriched rice milk and almond milk are a lot of lower in potassium, phosphorus and protein than bovine's milk, making them a decent substitute for milk while on a renal eating routine.

What to eat in a renal diet?

Eat a high protein nourishment at each supper. This incorporates meat, fish, poultry, new pork or eggs.

Cut out potassium and phosphorus.

Dodge nutty spread, nut, seeds, dried beans and lentils. Despite the fact that these are high in protein, they are additionally high in potassium and phosphorous.

Utilize less salt and eat less salty nourishments. This may control pulse and lessen weight gains between dialysis sessions.

Use herbs, flavors and low-salt flavor enhancers instead of salt

Maintain a strategic distance from salt substitutes made with potassium.

Evade entire grain and high fiber nourishments, for example, entire wheat bread, grain oat and dark colored rice as far as possible your admission of phosphorous.

Utmost your admission of milk, yogurt and cheddar. These are high in phosphorus. Constraining dairy-based nourishments ensures your bones and veins.

All organic products have some potassium. Constraining potassium secures your heart. Pick apples and berries over oranges and bananas.

All vegetables have some potassium. Pick broccoli and cabbage over potatoes and asparagus.

What you can drink in the renal diet?

Things you can drink

How much liquid and kinds of liquid your admission is significant for the constant kidney infection patient to screen. A few patients may have been asked by their doctor to screen as well as limit the measure of liquids they take in.

Your liquid admission ought to be observed by inspecting your individual liquid status. In the event that you are holding liquid, cut back on your admission and the other way around.

1. Individuals with sound kidneys should drink 8-10 eight-ounce glasses (64 ounces) of water ordinary

2. Patients on dialysis as well as patients experiencing a "wiped out period," may display indications of lack of hydration. Indications of lack of hydration include: migraines, indigestion, joint and back torment, kidney stones, clogging, exhaustion and dazedness.

3. Patients on diuretics might be progressively vulnerable to lack of hydration.

4. Drinking water brings down danger of urinary tract and bladder contaminations, which can be basic in kidney illness patients.

5. Indications of liquid over-burden incorporate swollen fingers and lower legs, hypertension, swelling and trouble relaxing.

Is liquor or soft drink awful for the kidneys?

Not generally. With some restraint, liquor and soft drink are not awful for the kidneys. Yet, both influence the kidneys in a roundabout way. Mixed refreshments and soft drinks are high in calories, and a lot of them are bad for anybody with diabetes. Diabetes is the main source of kidney disappointment. Likewise, while liquor influences the liver all the more straightforwardly, it can raise circulatory strain. What's more, cause lack of hydration. Hypertension may harm the kidneys.

Hypertension is the number two reason for kidney disappointment. Liquor likewise can be hazardous to drink when you are on certain sorts of medication. Try to get some information about how liquor can influence your medications.

Another investigation connected drinking at least two sugary beverages every day with an expanded hazard for hypertension.

Is cranberry squeeze useful for the kidneys?

Cranberry juice may help avoid urinary tract contaminations (UTIs). The juice makes it hard for germs (microscopic organisms) to develop in your bladder. In the event that you are inclined to UTI's as well as kidney contaminations, incorporating 100% cranberry squeeze in your day by day admission may be a smart thought.

Shouldn't something be said about caffeinated drinks?

Caffeinated beverages ought to be utilized with alert. They are soda pops whose makers promote that they support vitality. Most contain a wellspring of caffeine as their significant fixing. Interminable kidney sickness patients should screen the measure of caffeine that they incorporate into their weight control plans and limit it to under 200-mg/day. Allude to the rundown beneath for caffeine admission in like manner drinks and nourishment things.

Nourishment Item (Caffeine Content)

Blended Coffee (100mg)

Hershey's Milk Chocolate Kisses (5mg)

M&M's Milk Chocolate (16mg)

Mountain Dew (56mg)

Snapple Iced Tea (38mg)

Starbucks Coffee Frappuccino (166mg)

How much water would it be advisable for me to drink?

You should not have to drink eight glasses of water each day to remain sound, as once thought. Yet, water is as yet a superior decision than drinks that have caffeine like pop, espresso or tea. These beverages can really make you thirstier. Staying away from extra sugary squeezes and fruit juices is likewise a smart thought, particularly on the off chance that you have diabetes. Drinking a lot of water may likewise help avoid kidney stones. Continuously make a point to remain inside your doctor's liquid admission suggestions and watch for liquid over-burden.

Recipes

This chapter will throw light on various meals that have a renal ingredient in them

Breakfast

Dilly Scrambled Eggs

Ingredients

2 huge eggs

1/8 teaspoon dark pepper

1 teaspoon dried dill weed

1 tablespoon disintegrated goat cheddar

Supplements per serving

Calories 194

Protein 16 g

Starches 1 g

Fat 14 g

Cholesterol 434 mg

Sodium 213 mg

Potassium 192 mg

Phosphorus 250 mg

Calcium 214 mg

Fiber 0.2 g

Readiness

Beat the eggs in a bowl; empty them into a nonstick skillet over medium warmth.

Include dark pepper and dill weed to eggs.

Cook until eggs are mixed.

Top with disintegrated goat cheddar before serving.

Renal and renal diabetic nourishment decisions

2 meat

1 fat

Sugar decisions

Supportive insights

1/2 cup low cholesterol egg item can be substituted for 2 eggs for a lower fat and cholesterol dish. Cholesterol is diminished to 11 mg, fat 4 mg, and phosphorus 73 mg.

Cindy inclines toward The Pampered Chef® All-Purpose Dill Mix.

Substitute one tablespoon crisp dill for dried dill weed whenever wanted.

Speedy and Easy Apple Oatmeal Custard

Fixings

1/3 cup snappy cooking oats

1 enormous egg

1/2 cup almond milk

1/4 teaspoon cinnamon

1/2 medium apple

Supplements per serving

Calories 248

Protein 11 g

Sugars 33 g

Fat 8 g

Cholesterol 186 mg

Sodium 164 mg

Potassium 362 mg

Phosphorus 240 mg

Calcium 154 mg

Fiber 5.8 g

Planning

Center and finely slash apple half.

Join oats, egg and almond milk in a huge mug.
Mix well with a fork. Include cinnamon and
apple. Mix again until completely blended.
Cook in microwave on high for 2 minutes.
Lighten with a fork. Cook an extra 30 to 60
seconds if necessary. Mix in somewhat more
milk or water if more slender oat is wanted.

Renal and renal diabetic nourishment decisions

1 meat

1 starch

1 milk substitute

1 organic product, low potassium

Sugar decisions

2

Supportive clues

For extra flavor supplant ground cinnamon with finely ground stick cinnamon.

Cooking time may change for various microwaves.

Sprinkle oats with 2 teaspoons of nectar whenever wanted. Consider an extra 12 grams of starch and 1 sugar decision in the event that you pursue a starch tallying dinner plan for diabetes. Substitute 1/4 cup 1% low fat milk and 1/4 cup water for almond milk whenever liked. These progressions the protein to 12 grams, phosphorus to 278 mg and potassium to 358 mg.

Oats is higher in potassium and phosphorus contrasted with refined grains, however can be incorporated into most kidney abstains from food. Talk about with your dietitian on the off chance that you are uncertain.

Microwave Coffee Cup Egg Scramble

Fixings

1 enormous egg

2 enormous egg whites

2 tablespoons 1% low fat milk

1/8 teaspoon dark pepper

Supplements per serving

Calories 117

Protein 15 g

Starches 3 g

Fat 5 g

Cholesterol 188 mg

Sodium 194 mg

Potassium 226 mg

Phosphorus 138 mg

Calcium 72 mg

Fiber 0 g

Arrangement

Splash a 12-ounce espresso mug with cooking shower. Consolidate the milk, egg and egg whites in the mug and beat until mixed. Spot espresso mug in microwave and cook for 45 seconds; expel and mix. Microwave an expansion 30-45 seconds, until eggs are nearly set.

Sprinkle with pepper and appreciate.

Need increasingly heavenly kidney-accommodating plans like Microwave Coffee Cup Egg Scramble?

Smoothies and drinks

Blueberry Smoothie

Fixings

1 cup solidified blueberries

8 bundles of Splenda®

6 tablespoons of protein powder

8 ice 3D squares

14 ounces of squeezed apple (no additional sugar)

Supplements per serving

Calories 108

Protein 9 g

Starches 18 g

Fat 0 g

Cholesterol 0 mg

Sodium 27 mg

Potassium 183 mg

Phosphorus 42 mg

Calcium 57 mg

Fiber 1.2 g

Arrangement

Spot all fixings in a blender and mix until smooth.

Simple Pineapple Protein Smoothie

Fixings

3/4 cup pineapple sherbet or sorbet

1 scoop vanilla whey protein powder

1/2 cup water

2 ice 3D squares, discretionary

Supplements per serving

Calories 268

Protein 18 g

Starches 40 g

Fat 4 g

Cholesterol 36 mg

Sodium 93 mg

Potassium 237 mg

Phosphorus 160 mg

Calcium 160 mg

Fiber 1.4 g

Arrangement

In a blender, include pineapple sherbet, whey protein powder and water (ice 3D squares discretionary).

Promptly mix for 30 to 45 seconds.

Snacks and sides

Nibbling when you're on the kidney diet

Eating is alright on the kidney diet as long as you settle on solid decisions. As opposed to eating nourishment that is high in sodium, for example, a little sack of potato chips, a superior choice is a bit of kidney-accommodating organic product. You likewise need to think about the amount you eat by and large. Eating shouldn't be synonymous with blame. On the off chance that your doctor urges you to build your calorie admission, your renal dietitian will examine the best nibble decisions for you. Bites can compensate for low-calorie consumption when your hunger isn't so extraordinary.

Kidney-accommodating snacks at the supermarket

Experience any treat or wafer passageway of your neighborhood market and you'll locate a wide cluster of tidbits. In any case, on the off chance that you have CKD you should restrain or stay away from specific fixings that might be available in nibble nourishments. Your primary care physician or dietitian may prescribe that you limit your admission of phosphorus, potassium, sodium and calcium if your kidneys are never again ready to keep these minerals in balance. By instructing yourself and with the assistance of your social insurance group, there are numerous kidney-accommodating, sound and scrumptious snacks accessible. Go to the produce area where you can discover kidney-accommodating nourishments for a decent nibble choice. Here are a few nourishments useful for kidney wellbeing:

Apples

Blueberries

Carrot sticks

Fruits

Dried, improved cranberries

Grapes

Raspberries

Red ringer peppers

Red leaf lettuce

Strawberries

Lunch

Bar-b-que Chicken Pita Pizza

Fixings

2 pita breads, 6-1/2" size

3 tablespoons low-sodium grill sauce

1/4 cup purple onion

2 tablespoons disintegrated feta cheddar

4 ounces chicken, cooked

1/8 teaspoon garlic powder

Supplements per serving

Calories 320

Protein 23 g

Sugars 37 g

Fat 9 g

Cholesterol 55 mg

Sodium 523 mg

Potassium 255 mg

Phosphorus 221 mg

Calcium 163 mg

Fiber 2.4 g

Planning

Preheat broiler to 350° F.

Shower preparing sheet with nonstick cooking splash and spot 2 pitas on sheet.

Spread 1-1/2 tablespoon BBQ sauce on every pita.

Hack onion and spread over pitas.

3D square chicken and spread over pitas.

Sprinkle feta cheddar and garlic powder over pitas.

Prepare for 11 to 13 minutes.

Conclusion

To conclude the book, you have to be very careful about diet intakes that you do throughout your routine. You need to be curious about every calorie that goes in you. You have been provided with all the reasons in this book about the process of renal diet. Renal diet can give you a healthy ph and can avert any harmful stroke of acidity in the body. Acidity can be dangerous in profuse accumulation fats, rise to inflammatory disease, the rupture in many digestion organs and having a rusted metabolism that does not work in the flow. On the contrary, renal diet can give you a fresh intake of all healthy diets that can be very healthy and caring for you. These diets are present in all formats.

They are in breakfast recipes, the dinner recipes, the lunch recipes, the smoothies and the sweat desserts that can up-satisfaction in your mouth. You do not have to be an expert of medicine to know which diet to follow when. You just have to know the diet intake of your own body and see how you are able to cater to the plight of diseases. You must not be able to compound yourself with the attack of acidity but must have the courage to use these diets and recover at the earliest.

These diets have everything in their DNA. They have the minerals, the enzymes, the protein, the amino acids, and whatnot. Green refluxes along with curing liquids are present in these diets and they come in all whims and fancies of the diet expression. There is no rocket science behind their creation and one has to be very intelligent while creating them. You can also follow this book and will get a splendid amount of results in no time. It is available at an affordable price.

Try your best in avoiding any acidic diet at all cost even if it gives you a great amount of relish. The idea is fats and mineral are very delicious but they come with devious outcomes of fat accumulation and strengths.

You need to understand that long aging is only possible if you have a balanced diet intake and this diet can be only of an keto.

To make conclusive remarks of the book about the benefits of an renal diet, the first and foremost is the sheer activeness that a person tends to achieve while he is eating an renal diet. He feels healthy and looks healthy and wants to be doing a lot of things while he is having an renal diet. He can think properly and can get rid of inflammatory diseases that can cause him suffering. He has a strong discipline that can be navigated in any way possible and thus, he is the next big thing for his users. Also, the longevity of life in this scenario and truly, an renal diet can do a lot of wonders for the individual. Therefore, an renal diet has a lot to do for the fitness and active-ness in the human body.

Furthermore, If you want to look green and fresh on your face, then the renal diet can be very helpful in this regard. Studies show that the renal diet is very popular in making a healthy face for you. The number of herbs and breakfast recipes you have for yourself, up-bring a good amount of freshness on your face as well on your skin. Thus, renal diet is very crucial for having great skin and face.

An renal diet protects bone density and muscle mass. The mineral intake that you get after having an renal diet can protect your bone density. The bones need certain minerals that are used to cure the excessive number of hurdles one gets while running. The minerals are given by the renal diet and you are able to get a stronger bone for life. If you are a bodybuilder and want to reap the benefits of the bone then you have to accumulate more renal diet in you that can be very beneficial for you. The muscle mass can be secured in an acute manner if you tend to get more and more almonds and other renal dietaries. You have to be very lenient when you are having the renal diet because the benefit of an renal diet like the muscle mass and the bone density will be instrumental for you. Just always look at the bright side of the diet and you will feel very productive while you do it.

In today's world, tensions are like a haunting disease that wants to remain at your back for no reason. Everywhere you go, you get a tertiary level of tension. There is the tension of graduating, the tension of succeeding in life, the tension of getting a job and tension of whatnot. You believe that tension can be very successive for you but in the latter, it turns out to be adverse. Scientists have claimed very medical drugs for its cure but the only reasonable cure for are the use of an renal diet. The enzymes that you get through vegetables lower the risk of your hyper blood tension and then you can achieve all the relish of your lifestyle in no time. Also, your blood level starts to resonate with full capacity and you will feel like a superman every place you go, therefore; hypertension and tensed matters get an upper hand of resolution when you get to know the prospect of an renal diet.

You are able to get a lot of chronic pains in your body due to many reasons. You get to the bottom of any problem; you solve it and end up having chronic pain in your body. Chronic pain refers to any tertiary amount of pain in your body and you are able to get to the harmfulness of it in no time. Therefore, chronic pain is the most devastating headache that you can get and the only effective cure of it is the renal diet. Yes, the renal diet is very important for you to maintain as the blood level minimizes when lemon or other keto water is induced in the body. So, this is another benefit of an renal diet and it does not matter if you are a walker, a boxer or even a corporate worker, you must have an renal diet in you if you wish to give all that you crave.

In the end, we will only assure you good health and being a beginner, you must waste any further time and order this book in a jiffy.

Because health is wealth nobody became rich while being lazy and stubborn. This book is all that you need and you must get at all cost.